T0332243

Copper and Zinc in Inflammation

INFLAMMATION AND DRUG THERAPY SERIES
VOLUME IV

Copper and Zinc in Inflammation

Edited by

R Milanino
Institute of Pharmacology
University of Verona
Italy

KD Rainsford
Department of Biomedical Sciences
McMaster University Faculty of Health
Sciences
Hamilton, Ontario
Canada

GP Velo
Institute of Pharmacology
University of Verona
Italy

KLUWER ACADEMIC PUBLISHERS
DORDRECHT / BOSTON / LONDON

Distributors

For the United States and Canada: Kluwer Academic Publishers,
PO Box 358, Accord Station, Hingham, MA 02018-0358, USA
For all other countries: Kluwer Academic Publishers Group,
Distribution Center, PO Box 322, 3300 AH Dordrecht, The
Netherlands

British Library Cataloguing in Publication Data

Copper and zinc in inflammation.
  1. Man. Tissues. Inflammation. Role of copper & zinc
  I. Milanino, R. (Roberto) II. Rainsford, K. D. (Kim D.)
  1941– III. Velo, G.P. (Giampaolo), *1943–*
  IV. Series
616.07′2

  ISBN 0-7462-0079-X

Copyright

Published in the United Kingdom by Kluwer Academic Publishers,
PO Box 55, Lancaster, UK.

Kluwer Academic Publishers BV incorporates the publishing
programmes of D. Reidel, Martinus Nijhoff, Dr W. Junk and
MTP Press.

Printed in Great Britain by Butler & Tanner Limited, Frome and London

Contents

Preface

The role of trace metals, especially copper and zinc, in the pathogenesis of rheumatic conditions has continued to receive much interest following the initial upsurge of research activity in the 1970s. Meantime also copper and zinc complexes receive continued attention for their potential anti-inflammatory actions. Since the previous major titles were published in this field some years ago (e.g. 1,2) it was considered timely to consider progress which has been made in the interceding period. Thus in this volume aspects are reviewed of the metabolism and biodisposition of copper and zinc, especially as they may be influenced by inflammatory processes, the mode of action of copper and zinc compounds in inflammatory states, and the actions of some newer copper complexes. While we still understand relatively little about how copper and zinc complexes work in inflammation, and indeed what the fate of the ligands and their complexed ions is in inflammation, it is hoped that this volume will be useful for giving a current view of the "state of art" in the field.

Special thanks are given to the valued efforts of the contributors, Dr Peter Clarke (Publishing Director, Kluwer Academic Publishers) and Mrs Veronica Rainsford-Koechli for her help in proof-reading the manuscripts.

K D Rainsford
Hamilton, Ontario, Canada
February 1989

References

1. Rainsford, K.D., Brune, K. and Whitehouse, M.W. (eds) (1981). Elements in the pathogenesis a treatment of inflammation. (Basel: Birkhauser)
2. Sorenson, J.R.J. (ed) (1982). *Inflammatory Diseases and Copper.* (New York: Humana Press)

List of Contributors

L.M. BAMBARA
Istituto di Patologia Medica
Università di Verona
Policlinico Borgo Roma
37134 Verona
Italy

S.J. BEVERIDGE
Department of Applied Sciences
Hunter Institute of Higher Education
PO Box 84 Waratah NSW 2298
Australia

M. BRESSAN
Dipartmento di Chimica Inorganica
Metallorganica ed Analitica
Università di Padova
Centro CNR, via Marzollo 1
35131 Padova
Italy

E. CONCARI
Istituto di Farmacologia
Università di Verona
Policlinico Borgo Roma
37134 Verona
Italy

R.J. COUSINS
Food Science and Human Nutrition
Department
Center for Nutritional Sciences
University of Florida
Gainesville, FL 32611
USA

J.A. CUTHBERT
Department of Internal Medicine
University of Texas Southwestern
Medical Center at Dallas
5323 Harry Hines Boulevard
Dallas, TX 75235-9030
USA

C.W. DENKO
Rheumatology Division
Department of Medicine
Case Western Reserve University
Cleveland, OH 44106
USA

F. FERNANDEZ-MADRID
Department of Internal Medicine
Wayne State University School of
Medicine
Gordon Scott Hall of Basic Sciences
540 East Canfield Avenue
Detroit, MI 48201
USA

A. FRIGO
Istituto di Patologia Medica
Università di Verona
Policlinico Borgo Roma
37134 Verona
Italy

A. GRIDER
Food Science and Human Nutrition
Department
Center for Nutritional Sciences
University of Florida
Gainesville, FL 32611
USA

P.L. JEFFREY
Department of Internal Medicine
University of Texas Southwestern
Medical Center at Dallas
5323 Harry Hines Boulevard
Dallas, TX 75235-9030
USA

P.E. JOHNSON
United States Department of Agriculture
Agriculture Research Service
Grand Forks Human Nutrition Research
Center
PO BOX 7166 University Station
Grand Forks, ND 58202
USA

P.E. LIPSKY
Department of Internal Medicine
University of Texas Southwestern
Medical Center at Dallas
5323 Harry Hines Boulevard
Dallas, TX 75235-9030
USA

J. LUNEC
Department of Biochemistry
Selly Oak Hospital
Birmingham B29 6JD
UK

M. MARRELLA
Istituto di Farmacologia
Università di Verona
Policlinico Borgo Roma
37134 Verona
Italy

R. MILANINO
Istituto di Farmacologia
Università di Verona
Policlinico Borgo Roma
37134 Verona
Italy

U. MORETTI
Istituto di Farmacologia
Università di Verona
Policlinico Borgo Roma
37134 Verona
Italy

A. MORVILLO
Dipartmento di Chimica Inorganica
Metallorganica ed Analitica
Università di Padova
Centro CNR, via Marzollo 1
35131 Padova
Italy

K.D. RAINSFORD
Department of Biomedical Sciences
McMaster University Faculty of Health
Sciences
Hamilton, Ontario
Canada L8N 3Z5

J.R.J. SORENSON
Division of Medicinal Chemistry
University of Arkansas College of
Pharmacy
4301 W. Markham Street
Little Rock, AR 72205
USA

C. TAMBALO
Istituto di Patologia Medica
Università di Verona
Policlinico Borgo Roma
37134 Verona
Italy

G.P. VELO
Istituto di Farmacologia
Università di Verona
Policlinico Borgo Roma
37134 Verona
Italy

1
Copper and zinc in inflammation

CW Denko
Rheumatology Division
Department of Medicine
Case Western Reserve University
Cleveland, Ohio 44106, USA

I. INTRODUCTION

Inflammation is a desirable complex process by which the organism controls and repairs effects of noxious stimuli. Efficacy of the organism in ameliorating the undesirable effects of inflammation is measured by decreases in the four cardinal features of inflammation, pain, redness, heat and swelling, is with the ultimate aim of preventing loss of function. Experimental studies teach that copper and zinc are fundamentally involved in the expression and control of inflammation. How copper and zinc metabolism changes in inflammatory states and how inflammation modulates the organism's fluctuating copper and zinc levels are discussed using examples from laboratory experiments and from natural experiments such as rheumatoid arthritis.

II. EXPERIMENTAL STUDIES

Animals made deficient by restricting dietary copper and dietary zinc[1-3] react with increased inflammation when challenged by injections of carrageenan and by injections of monosodium urate crystals. Replenishment of deficient diets with copper and with zinc before challenge resulted in reduced inflammation. Injection and dermal applications of diverse copper compounds, e.g. caeruloplasmin, copper salts of amino acids, copper aspirinate and dietary zinc[1-3], into animals with experimental inflammation resulted in lessened inflammation[4-7]. Since hypercupremia is a common finding in inflammation why should adding more copper help control the inflammation? Probably it is not due alone to the level of copper which is responsible for therapeutic effectiveness but to the form of copper and its interaction with tissue proteins and trace metals. Exogenous copper given in treatment could re-establish endogenous copper equilibria. Copper forms an integral part of many

Copper and Zinc in Inflammation. Milanino, R, Rainsford, KD and Velo, GP (eds)
Inflammation and Drug Therapy Series, Volume IV

proteins as Cu^+ or Cu^{++} or both with shifts back and forth during enzymic action[8]. In the early inflammatory phase of adjuvant disease, five days after adjuvant administration, daily injections of zinc intraperitoneally stimulated serum caeruloplasmin and liver metallothionein production[9]. Serum copper levels also rose. Inflammation in the rat paw diminished when these biochemical changes took place.

How caeruloplasmin acts as an anti-inflammatory agent is difficult to isolate and may relate to more than one physiological function. Caeruloplasmin is an acute phase reactant and like other acute phase reactants increases in the inflamed organism. Caeruloplasmin action is influenced by environmental factors with the result that test comparisons are difficult especially when there are variations in proteins, metals, ascorbic acid, thiol groups and oxygen free radicals during testing[10]. The transport function of caeruloplasmin in carrying copper to needed sites is unlikely to account entirely for its anti-inflammatory action. In the cases of two other transport proteins which decrease during inflammation, namely albumin and transferrin, increases in their levels induce greater inflammation[11]. Caeruloplasmin has a local action which may relate to its enzymic or oxidase function since it is an effective anti-inflammatory agent when injected directly into the site of inflammation[6].

III. CLINICAL STUDIES

In rheumatoid arthritis, a common human form of inflammation, we find salient features of inflammation, pain, swelling, redness and heat, along with loss of function and perturbations of copper metabolism. With the advent of emission spectroscopy, Niedermeier and co-workers[12] undertook extensive studies of copper and other trace metals in patients with chronic rheumatoid arthritis. Mean serum concentrations of copper, molybdenum, manganese, tin, barium and cesium were elevated in rheumatoid patients when compared to normal controls. Zinc and iron levels were lower in rheumatoids than in controls. Copper levels rose following treatment with gold. Zinc and iron levels were not changed by treatment. Levels of two other essential trace metals: molybdenum and manganese, dropped after treatment as did levels of the non-essential trace metals: tin, barium and cesium.

A role for zinc in inflammation is suggested by this report of Niedermeier and co-workers showing serum zinc levels to be low in rheumatoid arthritis patients. Their zinc levels remained low after treatment, suggesting zinc levels may not be as accurate a measure of response as copper levels. Simkin[13] has reported zinc sulfate to be effective in improving patients with rheumatoid disease in Northwest USA. My experience in East Central USA in treating patients with rheumatoid arthritis with zinc sulphate does not indicate zinc to be effective in patients. Results were variable; some patients improved for a short time, then relapsed. In those that improved, improvement was gradual and not as pronounced as that occurring with other treatments. There may be differences in the degree of zinc deficiency between persons living in Northwest USA and East Central USA. Dietary intake may vary.

In studies of serum copper in another form of inflammation, ankylosing spondylitis, Pshetakovsky[14] reported copper levels to rise during the acute phase and to diminish with the chronic phase. Similar findings are noted in rheumatoid arthritis[15,16]. One of the mechanisms used to explain the protective action of copper compounds is the scavenging of oxygen-centred free radicals by the copper–zinc enzyme, superoxide dismutase[17] and by caeruloplasmin[6].

In the familial disorder known as Wilson's disease or hepatolenticular degeneration, perturbations of copper metabolism occur. Whether the disease actually begins in the liver or in the brain remains unsettled. Initially the liver fills with copper because of inadequate excretion via the biliary system; then the liver degenerates, slowly releasing copper that accumulates in brain and kidney. Usually serum copper and serum caeruloplasmin levels are low. Abnormal bony changes are common on X-ray. Premature osteoarthritis occurs with biopsies of symptomatic joints showing chronic inflammatory cell infiltrates. Removal of excess copper from the body is an effective treatment usually done by administration of penicillamine[18].

Table 1 Serum caeruloplasmin levels in normal men and normal women

Group	Age (years)	Number	Caeruloplasmin (mg/dl)	$p <$
Women	20–81	75	41 ± 13	0.002
Men	20–93	50	35 ± 8	

Based on data in Reference 19

Serum caeruloplasmin levels are higher in normal women than in age-matched normal men, Table 1[19]. Patients with common rheumatic disorders – rheumatoid arthritis, systemic lupus erythematosus (SLE), gout and osteoarthritis – show elevated caeruloplasmin along with changes in other acute phase proteins when compared with age- and sex-matched controls (Table 2)[20]. The greatest increases in caeruloplasmin occur in the patients with acute gout, the most severe inflammation. Usually these patients seek medical attention quickly after the onset of this urate-crystal-induced disorder. However, after the pain, redness, heat and swelling subside, the gout is controlled and enters the chronic phase. The serum caeruloplasmin drops to approach normal levels. Women who have higher normal values attain higher responses.

3

Table 2 **Serum caeruloplasmin in rheumatic disorders**

Group	Sex	Number	Average (age)	Caeruloplasmin (mg/dl)	p <
Rheumatoid arthritis	W	115	55	47 ± 15	0.01
Normal	W	76	47	41 ± 13	
Rheumatoid Arthritis	M	37	56	46 ± 13	0.01
Normal	M	40	50	36 ± 8	
SLE	W	38	43	48 ± 20	0.01
Normal	W	67	41	40 ± 13	
SLE	M	10	46	47 ± 8	0.00
Normal	M	37	37	33 ± 8	
Osteoarthritis	W	107	65	49 ± 18	0.02
Normal	W	41	54	43 ± 11	
Osteoarthritis	M	39	65	40 ± 12	0.07
Normal	M	32	58	36 ± 8	
Gout – acute	W	9	66	60 ± 13	0.01
Gout – chronic	W	20	62	49 ± 14	0.08
Normal	W	32	57	43 ± 11	
Gout – acute	M	16	57	50 ± 15	0.01
Gout – chronic	M	50	56	39 ± 14	0.09
Normal	W	43	50	36 ± 8	

Based on data in Reference 20

Caeruloplasmin is a fairly sensitive marker for inflammation since it increased significantly in women with osteoarthritis at a time when the transport proteins, albumin and transferrin, do not change significantly[20]. Although osteoarthritis encompasses inflammation in its constellation, the driving force is a metabolic one rather than an inflammatory action. The consensus on causes of osteoarthritis is that there is failure of cartilage repair. In women with rheumatoid arthritis and in women with SLE serum caeruloplasmin undergoes comparable increases. In men patients with rheumatic disorders increases in serum caeruloplasmin were more variable. Perhaps this may relate to the fact that men normally have lower values than do women.

In summary, investigators have demonstrated that endogenous copper, especially serum caeruloplasmin, rises during the acute phase of inflammation and falls during the chronic phase. Serum caeruloplasmin is a fairly sensitive indicator for inflammation. The more acute the inflammatory process in patients the greater is the increase in serum caeruloplasmin.

4

References

1. Denko, CW, Petricevic, M, Whitehouse, MW (1981). Inflammation in relation to dietary intake of zinc and copper. *Int J Tiss React*, **3**, 73–6

2. Milanino, R and Velo, GP (1981). Multiple actions of copper in control of inflammation: Studies in copper–deficient rats. In: Rainsford, KD *et al.* (eds), *Trace Elements in the Pathogenesis and Treatment of Inflammation. Agents and Actions*, Vol.8, (Suppl.), pp. 209–30

3. Milanino, R, Cassini, A, Conforti, A and Franco, L *et al.* (1986). Copper and zinc status during acute inflammation: Studies on blood, liver and kidneys metal levels in normal and inflamed rats. *Agents and Actions*, **19**, 215–23

4. Lewis, AJ (1978). A comparison of the anti-inflammatory effects of copper aspirinate and other copper salts in rat and guinea pig. *Agents and Actions*, 244–50

5. Denko, CW and Whitehouse, MW (1976). Experimental inflammation induced by natural occurring microcrystalline calcium salts. *J Rheumatol*, **3**, 54–62

6. Denko, CW (1979). Protective role of caeruloplasmin in inflammation. *Agents and Actions*, **9**, 333–36

7. Walker, WR (1982). The results of a copper bracelet clinical trial and subsequent studies. In: Sorenson, JRJ (ed), *Inflammatory Diseases and Copper*. (Clifton, NJ: Humana Press), pp. 469–82

8. Owen, CA Jr (1982). Biochemical aspects of copper-copper proteins, ceruloplasmin, and copper protein binding. Park Ridge, NJ, *Noyes Pub*, pp205

9. Cousins, RJ and Swerdel, MR (1985). Ceruloplasmin and metallothionein induction by zinc and 13-cis-retinoic acid in rats with adjuvant inflammation. *Proc Soc Exp Biol Med*, **179**, 168–72

10. Laroche, MJ, Chappuis, P, Henry, Y and Rousselet, F (1982). Ceruloplasmin: Experimental anti-inflammatory activity and physicochemical properties. In: Sorenson, JRJ (ed), *Inflammatory Diseases and Copper*. (Clifton, NJ: Humana Press), pp. 61–72

11. Denko, CW (1980). Phlogistic properties of the serum proteins, albumin and transferrin. *Inflammation*, **4**, 165–8

12. Niedermeier, W, Prillaman, WW and Griggs, JH (1971). The effect of chrysotherapy on trace metals in patients with rheumatoid arthritis. *Arth Rheum*, **14**, 533–538

13. Simkin, P (1976). Oral zinc sulfate in rheumatoid arthritis. *Lancet*, **2**, 539–42

14. Pshetakovsky, Il (1973). Pathogenetic role of trace elements (Cu, Ni, Mn) and their diagnostic value in ankylosing spondylitis (Bekterev's Disease). *Vop Rheum*, **13**, 17–20 (in Russian)

15. Bajpagee, DP (1975). Significance of plasma copper and ceruloplasmin concentration in rheumatoid arthritis. *Ann Rheum Dis*, **34**, 162–9

16. Scudder, PR, Al-Timini, D, McMurray, D *et al.* (1978). Serum copper and related variables in rheumatoid arthritis. *Ann Rheum Dis*, **37**, 67–70

17. McCord, JM (1974). Free radicals and inflammation: Protection of synovial fluid by superoxide dismutase. *Science*, **185**, 529–31

18. Owen, CR Jr (1981). Wilson's disease. The etiology, clinical aspects, and treatment of inherited copper toxicoses. Park Ridge, NJ, *Noyes Pubs*, pp. 215

19. Denko, CW, Gabriel, P (1981). Age and sex related levels of albumin, ceruloplasmin, $\alpha_1$antitrypsin, α_1-acid glycoprotein and transferrin. *Ann Clin Lab Sci*, **11**, 63–68

20. Denko, CW and Gabriel, P (1979). Serum proteins – transferrin, ceruloplasmin, albumin, α_1-acid glycoprotein, α_1-antitrypsin – in rheumatic disorders. *J Rheumatol*, **6**, 664–72

5

2

Copper proteins and their role as antioxidants in human inflammatory conditions.

J Lunec
Department of Biochemistry
Selly Oak Hospital
Birmingham B29 6JD, UK

I. INTRODUCTION

Redox (oxidation-reduction) reactions are ubiquitous in virtually all biochemical processes associated with human metabolism, and metals such as Fe, Cu, Mo, Mn, and Co have an essential role. Fe and Cu as transition metals are particularly suited to catalyse redox reactions, mainly because they possess labile d-electron configurations and thus have a range of accessible oxidation states enabling them to transfer electrons.

II. COPPER AND IRON AS PRO-OXIDANTS

Copper and iron have emerged during the evolutionary process as the two dominant metals involved in the reduction of oxygen to water. This process is fundamental to aerobic life and the basic mechanism by which we obtain energy. However, though both are essential elements for the functioning of many important enzyme systems, in high concentrations, and particularly when dissociated from carrier proteins, they are paradoxically highly toxic[1-3]. Both the toxicity and protection they confer relate to their reactivity with oxygen.

Oxygen is a powerful oxidant, yet it is kinetically inert. This paradox allows us to come to terms with oxygen in the atmosphere and control its use in essential biochemical processes. In order to survive we tread the fine line between activating oxygen sufficiently for reaction while at the same time ensuring that dangerous by-products are not allowed to propagate their adverse effects.

Oxygen has an almost unique electronic configuration - it has two

Copper and Zinc in Inflammation. Milanino, R, Rainsford, KD and Velo, GP (eds)
Inflammation and Drug Therapy Series, Volume IV

electrons located in its outer bonding orbital. Electrons find it energetically more favourable to pair if their spins are antiparallel, i.e. in the opposite direction. In the case of oxygen their spins are parallel and for energetic reasons kept apart. Oxygen with its two unpaired electrons seeks other electrons, and this need for electrons explains its oxidizing power. However, the one electron reduction of O_2 to superoxide $O_2^{\bullet-}$ is thermodynamically unfavourable, requiring a reducing couple of -330 mV. Transition metals such as Fe and Cu will react with O_2 in various ways by virtue of their labile d-electron configurations. If Cu or Fe salts are added to tissue slices or cultures they promote O_2 toxicity, while *in vivo* they are pressed into service as cofactors to control its reactions and destroy its dangerous by-products. An important agent of O_2 toxicity is thought to be the superoxide $O_2^{\bullet-}$ ion, which may be formed by the uncontrolled autoxidation of low potential cytochromes, iron-sulphur proteins and flavoproteins[4,5].

(1) The generation of superoxide during inflammation

During the process of inflammation, migratory neutrophils, eosinophils, or monocytes are stimulated by surface contact with foreign particulate matter, such as immune complexes, complement, superoxide itself or invading micro-organisms. Irrespective of whether particles are phagocytosed, surface stimulation causes the activation of an NADPH oxidase situated within the surface of the cell membrane. This enzyme provides the reducing potential for addition of one electron onto oxygen to generate $O_2^{\bullet-}$ during the respiratory burst[6-10].

Superoxide is a powerful reducing agent, capable of removing chelated Fe and perhaps Cu from their respective binding sites on proteins[11].

$$[M^{(n+1)+} \text{--- complex}] + O_2^{\bullet-} \rightarrow M^{n+} + O_2 + \text{complex}$$

Also $O_2^{\bullet-}$ will dismutate slowly to generate H_2O_2

$$O_2^{\bullet-} + O_2^{\bullet-} \rightarrow H_2O_2 + O_2$$

In the presence of reduced metal ions removed from protein complexes, H_2O_2 can then undergo Fenton reactions, as follows, to generate the highly reactive and destructive hydroxyl radical ($OH^{\bullet}$)

$$Fe^{2+} + H_2O_2 \rightarrow Fe^{3+} OH^- + OH^{\bullet}$$

similarly for Cu^+. In addition for Cu^{2+}

$$Cu^{2+} + H_2O_2 \rightarrow Cu^+ + 2H^+ + O_2^{\bullet-}$$

thus regenerating the $O_2^{\bullet-}$ anion.

The hydroxyl radical will react with almost all known molecules found in living cells, with an extremely high rate constant, in particular - amino acids, sugars, DNA bases, organic acids and phospholipids; i.e. almost anything at or close to its site of formation[12,13].

The reactivity of the hydroxyl radical relates to its ability to abstract an electron from a nearby molecule; however, by gaining an electron another radical species is created. One of the best examples of secondary radical reactions is the process of lipid peroxidation[14]. Biological membranes contain polyunsaturated fatty acids (PUFA) which possess methylene interrupted double bonds. The methylene position in PUFA is particularly sensitive to OH• attack resulting in hydrogen abstraction. The removal of H• from the PUFA in conjunction with oxygenation will result in peroxy radical formation (ROO•). This peroxy radical can then go on to react further by H abstraction and perpetuate this process, thus weakening and eventually destroying the cell membrane. Cu and Fe may also promote lipid peroxidation directly by decomposition of primary peroxides. Reduced complexes (e.g. Fe^{2+} and Cu^+) react with lipid hydroperoxides (LOOH) to give alkoxy radicals (LO•).

$$LOOH + Fe^{2+} (Cu^+) \rightarrow LO^\bullet + Fe^{3+} (Cu^{2+})$$

$$LO^\bullet + LH \rightarrow LOOH + L^\bullet$$

$$L^\bullet + O_2 \rightarrow LOO^\bullet$$

(2) Catalytic Cu and Fe in inflammation

Copper and iron have recently received considerable attention with regard to their presence in extracellular fluids in forms which can catalyse radical reactions[16,17].

Total plasma or serum copper has three principle forms. Caeruloplasmin (Cp), an α_2-globulin (which is elevated as an acute phase protein during inflammation) accounts for 80-90% of serum copper. The remaining non-Cp copper is present in equilibrium between albumin or small amino acid complexes. This non-Cp copper is also thought to be elevated during acute inflammation[19].

Lorber et al.[20] were the first to report a statistically significant elevation of serum copper concentrations in rheumatoid arthritis (RA) when these patients were compared with age-matched normal individuals. However, they found that almost the entire copper content could be attributed to that bound to serum caeruloplasmin, though discrepancies concerning the elevations of this copper in sera were attributed to differences in activity of the patient's disease. Later groups have established that copper is elevated in serum and also in the synovial fluid of RA patients[21,22]. However, the synovial fluid has been found by various workers to contain a proportionately larger amount of non-Cp bound copper[23]. It has been suggested that this non-Cp copper can also serve as a deleterious sulphydryl group oxidising agent[20].

9

$$2Cu^{2+} + membrane \Big\langle \begin{matrix} SH \\ \\ SH \end{matrix} \rightarrow 2Cu^+ + membrane \Big\langle \begin{matrix} S \\ | \\ S \end{matrix} + 2H^+$$

It has also been speculated that the beneficial effects of certain antirheumatic drugs such as pencillamine could be attributed to chelation of copper and promotion of its excretion[24].

The increase of synovial fluid (SF) copper was confirmed by Bonebrake et al.[25] and Scudder et al.[21,23] who found that, in addition to an increase in total serum copper, total SF copper from RA patients contained two components compared to only one in the synovial fluid from non-inflamed joints. The non-Cp component was tentatively identified as a Cu/albumin complex. The possibility that the latter results from proteolytic action during inflammation cannot be ruled out, however, since caeruloplasmin is proteolytically cleaved into several fractions, one a 60,000 Cu-containing fraction resembling albumin.

(3)   Measurement of catalytic iron and copper

Assays with the potential to measure copper or iron in a form capable of promoting free radical damage through the Fenton reaction have recently been described by Gutteridge and co-workers[16,17].

Gutteridge has developed assays which attempt to measure the availability of catalytic iron and copper complexes in the human body. Both methods are based on the catalytic degradation of DNA by the antitumour antibiotic bleomycin. Bleomycin will only degrade DNA in the presence of an iron salt, but in the case of the copper assay, bleomycin-dependent degradation of DNA will only occur when Cu is complexed with the chelating reagent 1,10-phenanthroline. Both methods require a suitable reducing agent such as ascorbic acid in the iron assay, or, in the case of the Cu assay, mercaptoethanol. Degradation of DNA results in production of thiobarbituric acid-reactive material (Abs 532 nm) which is the end-point measurement made in the assay.

The 'phenanthroline' assay detects copper bound to the high-affinity site of albumin and to histidine but not to caeruloplasmin. Copper ions attached to albumin and to amino acids may still interact with $O_2^{\bullet-}$ and H_2O_2 to form hydroxyl radical or some similar reactive species. Is the binding of Cu by albumin a biologically important mechanism for diverting low molecular weight Cu complexes away from binding to sensitive sites, e.g. cell membranes? $OH^\bullet$ production may be confined to the copper binding site, and because of the large amounts of albumin in sera, and particularly SF, this may be useful as a protective mechanism at sites of inflammation. In practice therefore copper-amino acid complexes may show up positive on the bleomycin assay but depending on the free radical generating system used such complexes may also have antioxidant activity and hence offset the inflammatory response. The addition of copper salt and hydrogen peroxide to proteins, in particular IgG, results in fluorescence formation and degradation of the protein[3]. Free radical degradation of IgG may be important in the pathogenesis of RA through the formation of immune complexes[26,27]. However, Cu histidine complexes resembling those thought to occur *in vivo* are not effective in stimulating IgG denaturation. Likewise copper salts have also been shown to degrade hyaluronic acid, the viscous lubricating component of synovial fluid, though again the relevance to copper complexes *in vivo* is questionable. One major criticism of the phenanthroline Cu assay is that caeruloplasmin is highly labile when separated from blood and undergoes proteolytic degradation under normal storage conditions (i.e. 4 °C, − 25 °C). Catalytic Cu may therefore be an artefact of long-term storage of specimens[29,30].

III. ANTIOXIDANT COPPER PROTEINS

Earlier in this chapter the concept of superoxide production from activated phagocytic cells during inflammation was introduced. McCord and others have shown that the pattern of degradation of hyaluronic acid observed in synovial fluid *in vivo* can be reproduced by exposing purified hyaluronic acid to an $O_2^{\bullet -}$ system *in vitro*[31,32]. This was the first evidence, albeit indirect, that implicated radical reactions in the aetiology of inflammatory joint disease. If these reactions occur during inflammation and cell activation how do we protect ourselves from such important physiological events? Paradoxically these reactions are controlled by important copper-containing enzymes which may have considerable antioxidant properties *in vivo*.

(1) Superoxide dismutase (SOD)

In 1969 McCord and Fridovich[33] clearly established that almost all oxygen metabolising organisms contain an enzyme which catalyses the dismutation of $O_2^{\bullet -}$ to hydrogen peroxide. These results were later confirmed by Bannister[34] and many others. SOD enzyme, previously known as erythrocuprein, was later renamed superoxide dismutase (SOD), and isolated from erythrocytes as the Cu–Zn form of the enzyme which is cyanide-sensitive and found in the cytosol: a second cyanide-insensitive copper manganese enzyme has been identified in mitochondria. Both enzymes appear to have identical specificities for superoxide anions, though it has been recently reported that superoxide dismutase may also react catalytically with peroxy radicals[35].

SOD catalyses most effectively the disproportionation of the superoxide radical by a mechanism that is presumed to involve the alternate reduction and oxidation of the copper ion at the active sites. There are two active sites which are thought not to interact with each other, and each contains 1Cu + 1Zn bridged by a histidine ligand. The Fe and Mn series of proteins are homologous in sequence but unrelated to the cupreins.

$$Cu^{2+} + O_2^{\bullet-} \rightarrow Cu^+ + O_2$$

$$Cu^+ + O_2^{\bullet-} \rightarrow Cu^{2+} + H_2O_2$$

$$\text{net effect: } 2O_2^{\bullet-} \xrightarrow{2H^+} O_2 + H_2O_2$$

(2) SOD and inflammation

The anti-inflammatory nature of the blue-green Cu-Zn SOD was discovered long before its enzymic nature had been detected. Palosein (a mixture of bovine SOD and sucrose) has been on the market since 1968, and has been shown by various workers to be an effective anti-inflammatory agent[36,37]. In tests on model inflammation systems, Palosein was shown to reduce swelling of the inflamed joint by 50% in 4 days as compared to a placebo which affected the same in 8 days. No clinically adverse effects were noted in 1000 patients despite a few allergic reactions which were reversible.

SOD is an enzyme whose synthesis can be induced. Exposure to increased concentrations of oxygen elicits increased synthesis of SOD. The same may be true of the inflammatory situation where $O_2^{\bullet-}$ is produced liberally. In an attempt to determine whether a deficiency of SOD can have some relation to disease process, several workers have shown that a diet low in copper enhances the inflammatory reaction in laboratory animals (for a review see ref. 38). This is in complete contrast to iron deficiency which inhibits inflammation[39]. Although, Rister has shown SOD to be deficient in the childhood form of rheumatoid arthritis[40]. In the adult form of the disease SOD levels in the intracellular compartment are **elevated** above those of age- and sex-matched controls[41]. This could be interpreted as an *in vivo* response to an increase in oxidative stress during inflammation.

(3) Extracellular superoxide dismutase

When McCord[31] first proposed that radical generation in the synovial compartment could have serious consequences for both the extracellular fluid and the connective tissue of the joint, he formed this hypothesis on the basis that there was little significant SOD activity in normal joint fluid. Hence, he suggested that a radical flux generated into the extracellular space would unleash its denaturing effects on biomolecules in an unprotected environment. Blake *et al.* have observed the SOD activity of synovial fluid in RA and reported it to be virtually non-existent, though other workers produce conflicting results[42,43].

12

Table 1 A comparison of major Cu-containing antioxidant enzymes in inflammation

	Superoxide dismutase	Caeruloplasmin	Extracellular SOD
Molecular wt	32,000 80,000	132,000	132,000.
Active centre	Cu/Zn (Mn)	Cu	Unknown
No. of active centre atoms	2/2(4)	6–8	4
Reactivity	$2 \times 10^9 \, M^{-1} \, S^{-1}$	$7 \times 10^5 \, MP^{-1} \, S^{-1}$	$1.25 \times 10^9 \, M^{1-} \, S^{-1}$
Location	cytosol mitochondria all cells	liver, blood	extracellular/ intracellular
Anti-inflammatory activity	Yes	Yes	Yes
Stability	Very stable	Labile	?Stable

Recently Marklund has observed a new type of SOD activity in extracellular fluids (EC SOD). This protein has now been isolated and purified. It has a molecular weight of 132,000 and contains 4 Cu atoms per mole of protein[44,45]. It has been found in all extracellular fluids including synovial fluids taken from patients with inflammatory joint disease, but as Table 1 shows it is many times less efficient at dismutating the $O_2^{\bullet-}$ anion than the intracellular enzyme. Marklund has investigated levels of EC SOD in rheumatoid synovial fluids versus age- and sex-matched osteoarthritic (non-inflammatory) fluid controls[46]. Controls had approximately twice as much SOD as synovial fluids: 63 ± 39 (U/ml) versus 29 ± 9 (U/ml) in a study of 15 in each group. One unit corresponds to 8.3 ng of human Cu Zn SOD. Plasma had a level of 20 units/ml. The results certainly indicate an insufficient level of protection within the environment of the inflamed joint, where levels of $O_2^{\bullet-}$ may reach the μmol range[47].

The extracellular space has very little protection against toxic products of oxygen reduction. In addition to a low SOD activity, the content of reduce glutathione is very low, and the catalase activity is negligible. Ascorbate has a high reactivity with the superoxide radical 2.7×10^5 mol $l^{-1} . \, s^{-1}$. Normal plasma concentrations of 50 μmol/l have sufficient capacity to remove $O_2^{\bullet-}$ but will be quickly oxidized in the process to dehydroascorbic acid. RA ascorbic acid levels are very low in the plasma and virtually absent in synovial fluids, particularly in fluid from inflammatory types of arthritis, suggesting increased oxidative stress in this disease[48].

(4) Caeruloplasmin: antioxidant activity

Caeruloplasmin is the blue-coloured copper-containing α_2-globulin of mammalian plasma. It has recently been identified as a single polypeptide with a molecular weight of 132,000 containing 6 or 7 copper atoms per molecule[18].

13

The copper in caeruloplasmin has been shown to exist in three distinct states: type 1 Cu^{2+}, which is responsible for the blue colour absorbing maximally at 610 nm (this absorbance is characteristic of tetrahedral complexes of Cu^{2+} with nitrogenous ligands such as histidine); type 2 which, like type 1, is paramagnetic but colourless; and type 3 which is not paramagnetic but absorbs at 330 nm. (Reviewed by Gutteridge and Stocks[18].)

(5) Ferroxidase activity

In vitro, caeruloplasmin catalyses the oxidation of a wide variety of polyamine and polyphenol substrates but, with the possible exception of bioamines, these oxidations have no known biological significance. Caeruloplasmin's biological role has been suggested to be that of a 'ferroxidase'[49,50]. This property may be linked to the incorporation of iron onto transferrin (by virtue of the oxidation of Fe^{2+} to Fe^{3+}). Caeruloplasmins oxidase activity is associated with an active centre involving histidine. It is thought to be, at least in part, by virtue of this activity that Cp can function as an extracellular antioxidant, inhibiting Fe^{2+}-catalysed reactions such as lipid peroxidation and the Fenton reaction[51-53] (Figure 1).

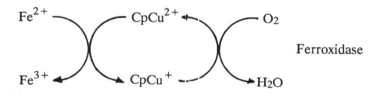

Figure 1 Inhibition of: (a) lipid peroxidation; (b) Fenton reaction

Caeruloplasmin therefore catalyses oxidation of Fe^{2+} and consequently produces a rapid four-electron reduction of molecular oxygen to water, with no intermediate formation of $O_2^{\bullet-}$ or peroxides. Stocks *et al.*[51] and Al-Timmini and Dormandy[52] found that the major antioxidant protein of serum was caeruloplasmin. Al-Timmini and Dormandy[52] further established that this antioxidant activity was related to caeruloplasmin's ability to inhibit the catalytic potential for oxidation of peroxidizing brain phospholipids. (It is worth noting here that in another system in which peroxy radicals are generated independently of iron, albumin is by far the most important antioxidant of human sera.)

(6) $O_2^{\bullet-}$ scavenging activity

A second important antioxidant activity of human caeruloplasmin is its ability to scavenge $O_2^{\bullet-}$ radicals. This property is a non-enzymic property and results in a stoichiometric reaction of Cp with $O_2^{\bullet -}$. It has been mistakenly cited as an SOD-like activity, but of course it is not. In contrast to SOD, caeruloplasmin reduced the yield of H_2O_2 expected from the dismutase reaction by almost 50%. The dismutation of $O_2^{\bullet -}$ by caeruloplasmin was only 1/3000 of that by SOD. Is Cp a significant scavenger *in vivo*, particularly during inflammation? The answer must be no, because to be an effective $O_2^{\bullet -}$ radical scavenger it needs to be available in excess of 200 mg/l [54]. The mean level of Cp present in 'inflammatory' types of fluids is 80 mg/l. However, at this level caeruloplasmin does provide considerable protection against iron-catalysed radical reaction due to its ferroxidase activity.

Table 2 In vitro models of free radical damage

Source of radicals	System	Damage	Protection
Hypoxanthine + Xanth ox	Cultured bovine articular cartilage	Synthesis of proteoglycans inhibited	Catalase protects
Hypoxanthine + Xanth ox	Human lymphocytes	Chromosomal damage, cell death	SOD catalase Desferrioxamine
Systemic activation of complement	Rat lung *in vivo* injury, death	Oedema cell Catalase	SOD
Cigarette smoke	α_1-antitrypsin	Partial inactivation	SOD Catalase
Hypoxanthine + Xanth ox	Infected into hind foot of rats	Oedema	SOD Catalase Mannitol
UV-irradiation activated neutrophils	IgG	Aggregation, antigenic, reactive with rheumatoid factor	SOD partial Catalase main Desferrioxamine
Hypoxanthine + Xanth ox	Collagen	Degradation, failure of gelation	SOD
Hypoxanthine + Xanth ox activated neutrophils	Hyaluronic acid	Depolymerization, loss of viscosity	SOD Catalase $OH^{\bullet}$ scavengers Metal chelators

Xanth ox = xanthine oxidase, SOD = superoxide dismutase

(7) Caeruloplasmin in Inflammation

Caeruloplasmin has been widely used as a measure of 'acute phase reactivity' in inflammation[55,56]. Like all other α_2-globulins it tends to be raised whenever there is active tissue damage. Though there is no specificity concerning the elevation of caeruloplasmin it is often quoted as being raised in rheumatoid inflammation. It has been postulated that caeruloplasmin is raised as are antiproteases by virtue of an increased synthesis during inflammation.

Table 3 Efficacy of SOD in inflammation

1.	Rheumatism - mainly oestoarthrosis	
2.	Conarthrosis	arthritis
3.	Coxarthrosis	
4.	Periarthritis	
5.	Epicondylitis	
6.	Rheumatoid arthritis	
7.	Chronic cystitis	
8.	Peyrone's disease	
9.	Lupus erythematosus	autoimmune
10.	Crohn's disease	
11.	Cardiac ischaemia/arrhythmias	

Elevated levels of copper and caeruloplasmin can be measured in both rheumatoid sera and synovial fluids; this has been confirmed by several workers[21,23,38,54]. Levels were always found to be higher in serum than in the corresponding fluid, and it was assumed that caeruloplasmin enters the site of inflammation in RA because of an increased permeability of the synovial membrane. However, one unconfirmed report by Gitlin and co-workers describes the ability of human synovial cells to produce caeruloplasmin *in vitro*[57]. Like α_1-antitrypsin and rat α_2-macroglobulin, caeruloplasmin has anti-inflammatory properties. Denko reported such activity against urate-induced rat paw oedema[58]. Previously when the observation was made that caeruloplasmin was elevated in synovial fluid from inflammatory joint disease, Scudder *et al.*[23] noted that there was a disproportionate amount of copper for the caeruloplasmin content of the fluid. The implications were that SF caeruloplasmin existed in at least two separate forms, one form possibly being induced by oxidation. Caeruloplasmin can be measured in at least two different ways: (1) by immunochemical assay using anti-human Cp antibody; (2) by virtue of its oxidase activity using either paraphenylene-diamine or Fe salt as substrate (ferroxidase assay)[59-61].

Previously we have measured both activities in synovial fluid in joint inflammation. We found[59] that the ferroxidase activity was disproportionately depressed relative to the amount of immunochemically determined Cp. This is in agreement with the results of Conforti *et al.*[62]. Their suggestion was that about 10% of caeruloplasmin contained in serum is present as the apoenzyme. However, we have shown that this disproportionate effect can be simulated by damaging caeruloplasmin using various forms of free radical generating system. We were thus able to impair the antioxidant activity of the protein by generation of $O_2^{\bullet-}$. This paradoxical effect would suggest that caeruloplasmin may have limited use as an antioxidant *in vivo* because it is easily damaged by $OH^{\bullet}$ radicals. Goldstein *et al.*[63] have shown that Cp itself scavenges $O_2^{\bullet-}$: $OH^{\bullet}$ may be produced in a site-specific manner on the metalloprotein. Oxidized biomolecules have been identified in a variety of pathological extracellular fluids, where free radicals are thought to be involved, and where caeruloplasmin would be expected to play a protective role[64,65]; for example oxidized α_1-antitrypsin in the serum of patients with emphysema and adult respiratory distress syndrome[66,67]. It is possible that the oxidation of these biomolecules may be secondary to the inactivation of antioxidants such as caeruloplasmin.

IV. SUMMARY

The toxicity of Cu and Fe in biological systems is intimately linked to the biochemistry of oxygen and free radicals. The reaction of biomolecules with oxygen is restricted because oxygen can receive electrons only one at a time. Transition metals such as Cu and Fe are found at the active sites of most oxidases and oxygenase enzymes, providing them with an efficient mechanism for accepting and donating electrons. This property allows them to overcome the spin restriction of oxygen. During inflammation we are protected from the onslaught of metal-catalysed free radical reactions paradoxically by antioxidant metalloenzymes such as superoxide dismutase and caeruloplasmin. Clearly, therefore, advancing our present knowledge about the anti-inflammatory effect of these copper-containing enzymes may lead to the therapeutic intervention of many diseases driven by inflammatory reactions which are 'out of control'.

REFERENCES

1. Gutteridge, JMC (1984). Iron-EDTA stimulated phopholipid peroxidation: a reaction changing from alkoxyl to hydroxyl radical dependant initiation. *Biochem J*, **224**, 697-701

2. Gutteridge, JMC and Wilkins, S (1983). Copper salt-dependent hydroxyl radical formation. Damage to proteins acting as antioxidants. *Biochem Biophys Acta*, **759**, 38-41

3. Phelps, Ra, Neet, KE, Lynn, LT and Putman, FW (1961). The cupric ion catalysis of the cleavage of gamma globulin and other proteins by hydrogen peroxide. *J Biol Chem*, 96-105

4. Harrison, PM and Hoare, RJ (1980). *Metals in Biochemistry*. (New York: Chapman & Hall)

5. Fridovich, I (1974). Superoxide dismutase. *Adv Enzymol*, **41**, 35-48

6. Roos, D (1977). Oxidative killing of microorganisms by phagocytic cells. *Trends Biochem*, **2**, 61-64

7. Fantone, JC and Ward PA (1975). Polymorphonuclear leukocyte mediated cell and tissue injury: oxygen metabolites and their relations to human disease. *Human Pathol*, **16**, 973-977

8. Ward, PA (1983). Role of toxic oxygen products from phagocytic cells in tissue injury. *Adv Shock Res*, **10**, 27-34

9. Babior, B (1984). Oxidants from phagocytes: agents of defense and destruction. *Blood*, **64**, 959-966

10. Segal, AW and Jones, OTG (1978). Novel cytochrome b system in phagocytic vacuoles of human phagocytes. *Nature*, **276**, 515-517

11. Halliwell, B (1978). Superoxide dependent formation of hydroxyl radicals in the presence of iron chelates. Is it a mechanism for hydroxyl radical production in biochemistry systems? *FEBS Lett*, **92**, 321-326

12. Halliwell, B and Gutteridge, JMC (1985). The importance of free radicals and catalytic metal ions in human diseases. *Molec Aspects Med*, **8**, 89-193

13. Lunec, J, Griffiths, HR and Blake, DR (1987). Oxygen radicals in inflammation. *ISI Atlas of Science: Pharmacology*, **1**, 45-48

14. Pryor, WA (1978). The formation of free radicals and consequences of their reactions in vivo. *Photochem Photobiol*, **28**, 787-801

15. Gutteridge, JMC (1986). Aspects to consider when detecting and measuring lipid peroxidation. *Free Rad Res Comm*, **1**, 173-184

16. Gutteridge, JMC (1984). Copper phenanthroline induced site specific oxygen radical damage to DNA. Detection of loosely bound trace copper in biological fluids. *Biochem J*, **218**, 983-985.

17. Gutteridge, JMC, Rowley, DA and Halliwell, B (1981). Superoxide dependent formation of hydroxyl radicals in the presence of iron salts. Detection of 'free' iron in biological systems by using bleomycin dependent degradation of DNA. *Biochem J*, **199**, 263-265

18. Gutteridge, JMC and Stocks, J (1981). Caeruloplasmin: physiological and pathological perspectives. *CRC Crit Rev Clin Lab Sci*, **14**, 257-329

19. Sterlieb, I, Sandson, JI, Morell, AG, Korotkin, E and Scheinberg, I (1969). Non caeruloplasmin copper in rheumatoid arthritis. *Arthritis Rheum*, **12**, 458-472

20. Lorber, A, Cutler, LS and Change, CC (1968). Serum copper levels in rheumatoid arthritis: relationship of elevated copper to protein alterations. *Arthritis Rheum*, **11**, 65-72

21. Scudder, PR, Al-Timmini, D, McMurray, W et al. (1978). Serum copper and related variables in rheumatoid arthritis. *Ann Rheum Dis*, **37**, 67-70

22. Youssef, AAR, Wood, B and Baron DN (1983). Serum copper: a marker of disease activity in rheumatoid arthritis. *J Clin Pathol*, **36**, 14-17

23. Scudder, PR, McMurray, W, White, AG and Dormandy, TL (1978). Synovial fluid copper and related variables in rheumatoid and degenerative arthritis. *Ann Rheum Dis*, **37**, 71-71

24. McMurray, W, Martin, WM, Scudder, P et al. (1975). Urinary copper excretion in rheumatoid arthritis. *Ann Rheum Dis*, **34**, 340-345

25. Bonebrake, RA, McCall, JT, Hunder, GC and Polley, HL (1968). Copper complexes in synovial fluid. *Arthritis Rheum*, **11**, 95-98

26. Lunec, J, Blake, DR, McCleary, S et al. (1985). Self-perpetuating mechanisms of immunoglobulin G aggregation in rheumatoid inflammation. *J Clin Invest*, **76**, 2084-2090

27. Lunec, J and Hill, C (1984). Some immunological consequences of free radical production in rheumatoid arthritis. In Borg, W et al. (eds), *Proceedings of the Third International Conference on Oxygen Radicals in Chemistry and Biology*, pp. 939-945. (Berlin: de Gruyter)

28. Niedermeier, W (1982). The effect of caeruloplasmin and iron on the L-ascorbic acid induced depolymerisation of hyaluronic acid. In Sorenson, JRJ (ed.), *Inflammatory Diseases and Copper*, pp. 223-229. (New York: Humana Press)

29. Gutteridge, JMC, Winyard, PG, Blake, DR et al. (1985). The behaviour of caeruloplasmin in stored human extracellular fluids in relation to ferroxidase activity, lipid peroxidation and phenanthroline detectable copper. *Biochem J*, **230**, 517-523

30. Winyard, PG, Pall, H, Lunec, J and Blake, DR (1987). Non-caeruloplasmin-bound

copper (phenanthroline copper) is not detectable in fresh serum or synovial fluid from patients with rheumatoid arthritis. *Biochem J*, **246**

31. McCord, J (1974). Free radicals and inflammation. Protection of synovial fluid by superoxide dismutase. *Science*, **185**, 529-531

32. Greenwald, RA and Moy, WW (1980). Effect of oxygen derived free radicals on hyaluronic acid. *Arthritis Rheum*, **23**, 455-463

33. McCord, J and Fridovich, I (1969). Superoxide dismutase: an enzymic function for erythrocuprein (Hemocuprein). *J Biol Chem*, **244**, 6049-6055

34. Bannister, JV (1973). The superoxide dismutase activity of human erythryocuprein. *FEBS Lett*, **32**, 303-306

35. Gee, CA, Kittridge, KA and Wilson, RL (1985). Peroxy free radicals, enzymes and radidation damage: sensititation by oxygen and protection by superoxide dismutase and antioxidants. *Br J Radiol*, **58**, 251-256

36. Cushing, LS, Decker, WE, Santos, FK *et al*. (1973). Orgotein therapy for inflammation in horses. *Mod Vet Pract*, **54**, 17-20

37. Lund-Olesen, K and Menander, KB (1974). Orgotein: a new anti-inflammatory metalloprotein drug. *Curr Therap Res*, **16**, 706-717

38. Milanino, R, Conforti, A, Franco, L *et al*. (1985). Copper and inflammation - a possible rationale for the pharmacological manipulation of inflammatory disorders. *Agents and Actions*, **16**, 504-513

39. Andrews, FJ, Morris, CJ, Kondratowicz, G and Blake, DR (1987). Effect of iron chelation on inflammatory joint disease. *Ann Rheum Dis*, **46**, 327-333

40. Rister, M, Bauermaster, IC, Gravert, U and Gladthe, F (1978). Superoxide dismutase deficiency in rheumatoid arthritis. *Lancet*, **1**, 1094

41. Youssef, AR and Baron, D (1983). Leukocyte superoxide dismutase in rheumatoid arthritis. *Ann Rheum Dis*, **42**, 558-562

42. Blake, DR, Hall, ND, Treby, DA *et al*. (1981). Protection against superoxide and hydrogen peroxide in synovial fluid from rheumatoid patients. *Clin Sci*, **64**, 551-553

43. Igran, I, Kaneda, H, Horiuchi, S and Ono, S (1982). A remarkable increase in superoxide dismutase activity in synovial fluid of patients with rheumatoid arthritis. *Clin Orthop Rel Res*, **162**, 282-287

44. Marklund, SL, Holme, E and Hellner, L (1982). Superoxide dismutase in extracellular fluids. *Clin Chim Acta*, **126**, 41-51

45. Marklund, SL (1982). Human copper containing superoxide dismutase of high molecular weight. *Proc Natl Acad Sci USA*, **79**, 7634-7638

46. Marklund, SL, Bjelle, A and Elmquist, LG (1986). Superoxide dismutase isoenzymes of the synovial fluid in rheumatiod arthritis and in reactive arthritides. *Ann Rheum Dis*, **45**, 847-885

47. Lunec, J, Wakefield, A, Brailsford, S and Blake, DR (1986). Free radical altered IgG and its interaction with rheumatoid factor. In Rice-Evans, C (ed.), *Free Radicals, Cell Damage and Disease*, pp. 241-261. (London: Richeliu Press)

48. Lunec, J and Blake, DR (1985). The determination of dehydroascorbic acid and ascorbic acid in the serum and synovial fluid of patients with rheumatoid arthritis (RA). *Free Rad Res Comm*, **1**, 31-39

49. Huber, CT and Frieden, E (1970). Substrate activation and the kinetics of ferroxidase. *J Biol Chem*, **245**, 3973

50. McKee, D and Freiden, E (1971). Binding of transition metal ions by caeruloplasmin (ferroxidase). *Biochemistry*, **10**, 3880

51. Stocks, J, Gutteridge, JMC, Sharp, RJ and Dormandy, TL (1974). The inhibition of lipid autoxidation by human serum and its relationship to serum proteins and alpha tocopherol. *Clin Sci*, **47**, 223-233

52. Al-Timmini, DJ and Dormandy, TL (1977). The inhibition of lipid autoxidation by human caeruloplasmin. *Biochem J*, **16**, 283-288

53. Lovstad, RA (1980). The protective action of caeruloplasmin on Fe^{III} stimulated lysis of rat erythrocytes. *Int J Biochem*, **13**, 221-224

54. Lunec, J, Wickens, DG, Graff, TL and Dormandy, TL (1982). In Sorenson, JRJ (ed.), *Inflammatory Diseases and Copper*, pp. 231-241. (New York: Humana Press)

55. Scheinberg, IH and Sternlieb, I (1960). Copper metabolism. *Pharmacol Rev*, **12**, 355

56. Rice, EW (1960). Correlation between serum copper caeruloplasmin activity and C-reactive protein. *Clin Chim Acta*, **5**, 632

57. Gitlin, JD, Gitlin, JI and Gitlin, D (1977). Localisation of C-reactive protein in synovium of patients with rheumatoid arthritis. *Arthritis Rheum*, **20**, 1491

58. Denko, CW (1979). Protective role of caeruloplasmin in inflammation. *Agents and Actions*, **9**, 333-336

59. Winyard, PG, Lunec, J, Brailsford, S and Blake, DR (1984). Action of oxygen free radical generating systems upon the biological and immunological properties of caeruloplasmin. *Int J Biochem*, **16**, 1273-1278

60. Sunderman, FW and Nomoto, S (1970). Measurement of human serum caeruloplasmin by its p-phenylenediamine oxidase activity. *Clin Chem*, **16**, 903-910

61. Buffone, CJ, Bret, EM, Lewis, SA *et al.* (1979). Limitations of immunochemical measurement of caeruloplasmin. *Clin Chem*, **25**, 749-751

62. Conforti, A, Franco, L, Milanino, R *et al.* (1982). Copper and caeruloplasmin activity in rheumatoid arthritis. *Adv Inflam Res*, **3**, 237-244

63. Goldstein, IM, Kaplan, HB, Edelsson, HS and Wiessmann, G (1979). Caeruloplasmin: a scavenger of superoxide radical anions. *J Biol Chem*, **254**, 4040-4045

64. Lunec, J and Dormandy, TL (1979). Fluorescent lipid peroxidation products in synovial fluid. *Clin Sci*, **56**, 53-59

65. Lunec, J, Halloran, SP, White, AG and Dormandy, TL (1981). Free radical oxidation (peroxidation) products in serum and synovial fluid in rheumatoid arthritis. *J Rheumatol*, **8**, 233-245

66. Carp, H, Miller, F, Hoidal, JR and Janodd, A (1982). Potential mechanism of emphysema: α1-proteinase inhibitor recovered from the lungs of cigarette smokers contains oxidised methionine and has decreased elastase inhibitory capacity. *Proc Natl Acad Sci USA*, **79**, 2041-2045

67. Cochrane, CG, Spragg, R and Revak, SD (1983). Pathogenesis of the adult respiratory distress syndrome. Evidence of oxidant activity in broncho-alveolar lavage fluid. *J Clin Invest*, **71**, 754-761

3
Role of metallothionein in copper and zinc metabolism: special reference to inflammatory conditions

A Grider Jr and RJ Cousins
Food Science and Human Nutrition Department
and Centre for Nutritional Sciences
University of Florida
Gainesville, Florida, USA

I. INTRODUCTION

There is an increasing body of evidence which suggests that in mammals copper and zinc metabolism is subject to hormonal regulation. The specific hormones involved include those that control key pathways of intermediary metabolism, e.g. glucocorticoids, glucagon, insulin and catecholamines. Furthermore, hormonal factors associated with the host defence system, e.g. interleukin-1, have similar regulatory effects. A significant factor in the regulation of these metabolic effects is directly related to control of metallothionein gene expression. In this brief review we will describe aspects of the metabolism of both trace elements as related to metallothionein as a functional entity, and how this is influenced by inflammatory conditions.

II. GENERAL CHARACTERISTICS OF METALLOTHIONEIN

Metallothionein (MT) has been characterized as a low molecular weight zinc- and copper-binding protein which functions in the homeostasis of these trace metals. The protein has been isolated from numerous species. Its amino acid sequence is highly conserved, which points to an important structure–function relationship. The occurrence of MT in both plant and animal phyla demonstrates its primitive evolution. MT has been found in all mammalian tissues assayed to date. However, the liver, kidney, and intestine appear to have the highest concentrations. Two major isoforms of MT are produced in most species. Separate genes control the production of these isoforms, which have been designated MT-1 and MT-2. Subforms have been identified in tis-

Copper and Zinc in Inflammation. Milanino, R, Rainsford, KD and Velo, GP (eds)
Inflammation and Drug Therapy Series, Volume IV

sues of some species, particularly humans. Nevertheless, MT-2 usually comprises the major form. MT concentrations in cells or tissues can be estimated by gel filtration and ion-exchange chromatography or measured by Cd^{2+} saturation, radioimmunoassay or ELISA methods. MT has been the subject of extensive reviews[1-5].

Mammalian MT contains 61 amino acids and has no histidine or aromatic amino acids. Twenty of the 61 amino acids are cysteine residues. However, all 20 are fully titratable with silver or 5,5'-dithiobis-(2-nitrobenzoic acid) indicating the absence of disulfide bonds[1]. MT is divided into two distinct metal-binding domains[6]. Domain A is the carboxyl half of the molecule representing amino acids 30 to 61. This domain contains 11 cysteine residues and binds four atoms of zinc, cadmium, or mercury (or six copper atoms). This half is resistant to EDTA metal chelation and subtilisin proteolysis. Domain B is the amino-terminal end of the molecule. This domain contains nine cysteine residues and binds three metal atoms of zinc, cadmium, or mercury (or six copper atoms). This half is the more labile portion of MT and is susceptible to EDTA metal chelation and subtilisin degradation[6,7]. The β domain may be more reactive for physiological aspects of MT since it exhibits greater ligand exchange. Metal exchange reactions can occur on the order of minutes[8].

MT exhibits binding affinities to elements from Groups I through V, and 22 of the transition elements[1,3]. Various procedures have been employed to determine the ranking of affinities which MT has for metals. There is a direct correlation between binding affinity and pH[9]. Those metals with a higher binding affinity dissociate from MT at a lower pH. The following order of binding affinities have been reported: Hg, Pd, Pt > Bi > Ag > Cu > Cd > In, Sb, Pb, Ru > Zn > Os > Ni > Co, Furthermore, these results are in agreement with established association constants published for metals and cysteine[10]. From a physiological perspective, only copper and zinc are relevant to normal cellular processes. Cu(I) binds in trigonal geometry with an affinity that is 10^5 times greater than the tetrahedral binding of Zn(II). However, on a particular basis zinc appears to be the most abundant metal associated with the protein except in fetal liver and adult kidney where significant amounts of copper and cadmium, respectively, are found[1].

1. Metallothionein inducibility by metals

A hallmark of interest in MT has centred on its unique, multifaceted inducibility. Regulation of MT gene expression is of particular significance because it is induced by metals which it in turn can tenaciously bind. Transcriptional control appears to account for most, if not all, of MT inducibility associated with metals[11]. This has been reviewed in detail[3,4]. Structural MT genes contain specific nucleotide sequences in the promoter region, viz. metal regulatory elements (MRE), that exist as multiple copies upstream from the TATA box and exert metal inducibility[12]. The most effective MRE sequence is

CTCTGCACTCCGCCCGA. A conserved MRE core $TGC_A{}^GC$ is necessary for metal regulation. How the MREs are able to exert their action is not clear, but it appears that trans-acting factors (presumably proteins) are able to interact with specific metal atoms that induce MT and then bind to the MRE sequence to allow transcription to proceed. Without a bound metal the factor(s) may act as a repressor. Within this conceptual framework it is understandable how MT is expressed to a greater extent in some tissues than others. Furthermore, manipulation of these factors or the genes that control them, could have significant therapeutic potential.

Under experimental conditions, administration of zinc, copper and other metals has been shown repeatedly to induce MT. The normal steady-state levels of the protein can be raised by orders of magnitude following acute or chronic administration of these metals to intact animals[1-5]. The level of MTmRNA is increased as the result of enhanced transcription rates[11]. Accumulation of the inducing metal accompanies increased synthesis[13]. Repletion of a dietary deficiency of zinc by refeeding can also produce marked increases in MT gene expression[14,15]. Recently, using oligonucleotide probes for the gene, MTmRNA levels observed in rats (fed purified diets with normal levels of zinc and copper) were higher in certain tissues compared to levels found when lower dietary levels were fed[16]. This suggests that MT structural genes in some tissues are normally expressed above basal levels under normal dietary conditions.

2. Metallothionein inducibility by hormones

Various types of stress increase hepatic MT levels[17]. Rats administered inflammation-producing agents, e.g. turpentine[18] or isopropanol[19] exhibit increased MT synthesis. The latter was shown to be correlated to increased MTmRNA. The effector molecules for MT induction by stress and organic molecules are probably activated by hormones rather than shifts in cellular metal content[2]. Glucocorticoid hormones increase zinc uptake by isolated hepatocytes via a process that increases cellular retention but not turnover[20,21]. Similarly, glucocorticoid administration increases MTmRNA and total MT levels in the liver[22]. The rate of transcription increases 90-fold over control levels within 2 h after administration of the hormone[23]. The promoter region for the glucocorticoid hormones has been identified and the DNA sequence of the MT-2 promoter region has been determined[24]. In human subjects glucocorticoid therapy significantly alters the kinetics of plasma to hepatic zinc transfer[25]. This response occurs in a fashion which suggests that hepatic uptake is subsequent to MT induction in response to therapy. In view of the use of glucocorticoid hormones as agents to treat specific disorders, including inflammation, the MT-linked effects it produces may explain some of the beneficial effects of therapy.

Evidence from data on a variety of inducible proteins demonstrates that multihormonal regulation is frequently involved. Food restriction is suf-

23

ficient to cause MT induction[26,27]. Given the nature of the complex hormonal factors involved in fasting, hormonal control is the most likely explanation for the induction. Glucagon, epinephrine and the intracellular mediator cAMP were tested for their effects on MT gene expression[28]. Each agent produced an increase in the number of MTmRNA molecules per hepatocyte and total liver MT. Of particular relevance was the finding that depression of serum zinc concentration was inversely related to hepatic MT levels. Subsequent kinetic data have shown that when hepatic MT is induced by dibutyl cAMP, as shown by elevated MT gene transcription, the transfer of zinc (^{65}Zn) from the plasma to liver MT is increased[29]. Experiments at the cellular level have been shown a classical gluconeogenic type of regulation for MT, viz, glucagon stimulates, but insulin inhibits, the response[30].

Acute infection has been shown to increase hepatic levels of both MT-1 and MT-2 concomitantly with hypozincaemia[31]. Depending on the infectious agent, *Salmonella typhimurium* (severe) or *Francisella tylanensis* (mild), the apparent half-life was altered 19 h vs. 38 h, respectively. Those rates of degradation agree favourably with those calculated from data with zinc-induced MT[32]. In the hamster, *E. coli* endotoxin administration produces marked depressions in serum zinc and elevated hepatic liver zinc concentrations within 4 h of administration. Liver copper did not change but serum copper exhibited a biphasic response with peaks at 8 h and 72 h after endotoxin[33]. This appeared to reflect changes in serum caeruloplasmin. The decline in liver zinc paralleled MT half-life. Maximum MTmRNA was observed 6 h after endotoxin, which places the induction sequence within the same time frame as observed with metals or glucocorticoid hormones. Injection with endotoxin from *Bacteroides melaninogenicus* prepared from dogs with gingivitis, had a greater effect on stimulation of serum copper and copper content of gingival tissue and less of an effect on hepatic MT than *E. coli* endotoxin. These findings suggest that different endotoxins may have differential tissue responses with respect to liver MT and zinc and copper metabolism during acute infection and subsequent inflammation.

Acute endotoxaemia and turpentine-induced inflammation are accompanied by increases in circulating glucagon[34]. It was proposed that glucagon is a factor that accounts for the MT-related changes in zinc metabolism. As described above, glucagon and the intracellular mediator of its action, cAMP, are able to elevate MT gene expression to a sufficient degree to produce hypozincaemia. Hepatic MT and MTmRNA levels increased by 10 h following the administration of dibutyl cAMP, epinephrine or glucagon to levels compared to those found with endotoxin[28]. In adrenalectomized animals these agents were less effective. However, they regained their potency when administered along with dexamethasone. In contrast, endotoxin-induced synthesis of MT was found to be independent of glucocorticoid regulation in transgenic mice[35]. These mice carry a fusion gene where the mouse MT-I promoter is linked to the Herpes simplex virus thymidine kinase structural gene. This fusion gene responds to heavy metal administration but not to glu-

24

cocorticoid hormones. Injection of endotoxin induced thymidine kinase to a level comparable to cadmium administration in these mice. Based on the results of DiSilvestro and Cousins[36], however, the hepatic MT in the transgenic mice may be responding to endotoxin-induced glucagon secretion or to other factors that increase cellular cAMP.

Endotoxin-induced changes in zinc metabolism are mimicked by interleukin-1 (IL-1). Administration of IL-1 causes a depression of serum zinc levels and increases in liver zinc MT[36–38]. IL-1 causes increased accumulation of zinc into the liver and spleen of mice[39]. Furthermore, the incubation of cultured human cells[40] (including kidney and liver tumour cells) with IL-1 increases the expression of the human MT-2_A. It is interesting that only the MT-2_A gene exhibited expression. In this cell line significant amounts of MT-1_A mRNA were not produced following IL-1 incubation. Human IL-1α produced by recombinant technology[41] stimulates MT production in intact rats (unpublished results). This IL-1 preparation contains the carboxyl-terminal 154 amino acids of the complete protein (271 amino acids). The temporal relationship is such that depression of the serum zinc concentration occurs concomitantly with elevation of MTmRNA and a 3-fold increase in total MT, but well in advance of the eventual 9-fold increase in liver MT. Both the spleen and kidney respond markedly to IL-1α and produce significant amounts of MT[38]. The serum zinc concentration became depressed and the liver zinc concentration increased following endotoxin injection into turkey embryos[42].

3. Metallothionein and metal metabolism

Hormonally regulated changes in cellular MT levels appear to involve zinc rather than copper[2]. Williams has proposed that, given a choice of appropriate ligands, cells should discriminate in descending order of preference $Cu > Zn > Ni > Co > Fe > Mn > Mg > Ca$[43]. Therefore, if zinc is to be utilized, the effect of copper binding must be minimized. This is probably accomplished through the incorporation of copper into apocaeruloplasmin. During inflammation this process is increased through the hormonal regulation of caeruloplasmin synthesis/secretion by hepatocytes[44].

Cellular zinc uptake/exchange has been characterized for hepatocytes. The turnover of zinc was about 15 h, suggesting that some ligands exhibit very rapid exchange rates[21]. Saturability of uptake is at the normal plasma zinc concentration, 9.5 μM, and the maximum exchange rate is 9.9 pmol Zn $\cdot$ min^{-1} $\cdot$ mg protein^{-1}. To drastically alter the plasma zinc pool new zinc binding sites need to be generated. When hepatocytes are stimulated with glucocorticoid uptake/exchange is increased, probably because efflux is reduced, thus favouring uptake rather than the exchange process. It is highly likely that all cells in which MT genes are expressed will respond to appropriate inducers and influence zinc metabolism in the intact animal. Analogous experiments suggest that copper metabolism in hepatocytes involves a balance between binding to MT and incorporation into apocaerulo-plasmin[44,45]. Cellular copper uptake/exchange also involves binding to MT but, at normal levels of exchangeable copper in plasma, considerably more zinc than copper would be expected to be transported into hepatocytes and bound to MT.

Kinetic experiments to measure changes in zinc and copper metabolism during the inflammatory process have not been conducted. These are essential, however, for a full appreciation of how metabolic fluxes of these elements are altered during inflammatory disease. Stimulation of MT gene expression with Bt$_2$cAMP produces a significant shift in the rate constant for transfer of zinc from the plasma to liver compartments[29]. The increase in hepatic uptake is accompanied by an increase in uptake by the bone marrow. Other metabolic compartments were not significantly affected by cAMP. The metabolically active nature of zinc in bone marrow is of interest because of the ability of the resident reticulum cells to remove toxins, and act as precursors for leukocytes. The expression of MT in the marrow progenitor cells has recently been demonstrated (unpublished data).

III. FUNCTIONAL IMPLICATIONS OF METALLOTHIONEIN RELATED TO INFLAMMATION

The well-documented regulation of metallothionein gene expression suggests that an important consideration for function rests on the ability of cells to rapidly produce large amounts of the protein. All potential functions of the protein could use that characteristic to advantage. From the standpoint of inflammatory disease, MT-related redistribution of copper and zinc between organs or within cellular compartments is its most likely role. This should be considered as host defensive in nature. A hypothetical scheme showing the integration of metallothionein in inflammation and its regulation is presented in Figure 1.

Donation of copper and zinc to apometalloenzymes is a logical function of the protein. This could be extended to include all metalloproteins that require copper or zinc. Experiments designed to demonstrate ligand exchange of copper or zinc to the apoprotein must be interpreted with caution. An equilibrium will be established between any apoprotein and an appropriate donor molecule, e.g. MT. Nevertheless, within cells the particularly high binding constant of MT for both copper and zinc, 10^{19} to 10^{17} and 10^{14} to 10^{11}, respectively[3], may provide a controlled transfer of metal atoms into specific proteins or other components providing ligands. Of recent interest relative to inflammation was the *in vitro* evidence showing that MT donates Cu(I) to apocaeruloplasmin when mediated by activated leukocytes[46]. This is supported by evidence in rats showing that induction of caeruloplasmin and reduction in acute adjuvant inflammation by 13-cis-retinoic acid is accompanied by increased liver MT[47].

26

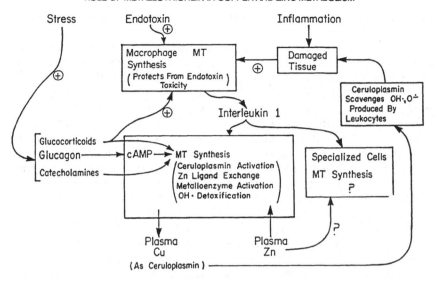

Figure 1 Hypothesis for the roles of metallothionein in inflammation.Bacterial infection and subsequent release of endotoxin (lipopolysaccharide) stimulate leucocytes. Monocytes are transformed into macrophages and invade the area of injury (contribution to inflammation) and secrete interleukin-1. This lymphokine stimulates metallothionein gene expression in many cells. This action may be direct or may require the combined effect of glucagon, glucocorticoids and/or catecholamines. Glucocorticoids also stimulate macrophages to produce metallothionein, which protects them from endotoxin toxicity. In the liver acute-phase proteins are induced, including caeruloplasmin and metallothionein. By donating zinc and copper, metallothionein may affect aproprotein activation. Caeruloplasmin is secreted into the circulation, resulting in increases in serum Cu. Hormonally stimulated metallothionein synthesis in the liver results in increased zinc binding and decreased serum zinc. The protein scavenger may detoxify free radicals in liver cells. Caeruloplasmin detoxifies free radicals at the site of injury. The effectiveness of treatment for chronic inflammatory disease may be influenced by control of metallothionein induction.

Cells with elevated MT levels appear to be able to resist a variety of stresses. The presence of MT in root systems of plants and in the gastrointestinal tracts of animals suggests that limitation of entry of heavy metals into other organ systems is a function of MT. As has been reviewed elsewhere, cells that lose the ability to produce MT are very sensitive to heavy metals[4]. Conversely, cells that over-produce MT are more resistant to specific metals than their counterparts that express MT genes normally. With intact animals, susceptibility to copper toxicosis, inherited or dietary, is also related to the ability to produce MT. Degradation of MT is directly related to the species of metal bound. Since MT containing copper is virtually undegraded it appears to accumulate in lysosomes as polymeric MT. Bound zinc appears to be removed from the protein during degradation as amino acids are returned to the cellular supply for reutilization[2]. It should be emphasized that while metals have differing rates of removal during degradation of the protein, ligand exchange reactions involving these metals occur for the entire life of the metalloprotein.

There is an increasing body of evidence that links the nutrient metals copper, iron and zinc to specific disease processes including inflammation. These areas have been reviewed in detail by Willson[48] and Halliwell and Gutteridge[49]. Briefly, Fe(II) is believed to participate in Fenton's reaction (Fe^{2+} + $H_2O_2 \rightarrow Fe^{3+}$ + OH^- + $OH^•$). H_2O_2 is produced in cells through superoxide dismutase activity. Cu(I) can substitute for Fe(II) in Fenton's reaction. However, within cells this potentially deleterious property of copper is limited or prevented through binding to MT and removal from liver cells as caeruloplasmin. The latter has demonstrated superoxide radical scavenging activity[50]. Dietary copper deficiency may contribute to inflammation because of a loss of this free radical scavenging activity of caeruloplasmin[51]. Nevertheless, production of superoxide radicals is a characteristic of activated neutrophils and macrophages, and is essential for destruction of evading bacterial cells and foreign substances. Induction of MT at a time when this host defence activity is maximised has a number of potential contributing functions that have a teleological basis of support. As will be discussed below, MT could: (1) stabilize cells from the hostile conditions produced, (2) contribute to activation of specialized cells and/or (3) act as a free radical scavenger.

The ability of cells to withstand metal toxicity after MT induction has been discussed above. However, MT induction is correlated to resistance to other conditions as well. Cultured cells that are stimulated with cadmium to produce large amounts of MT are resistant to platinum, gold and X-ray or UV radiation[52–55]. X-Irradiation and administration of gold to intact rats induces MT[56,57]. Pretreatment with zinc increased the binding of gold to MT[58]. This aspect of MT induction could limit the effectiveness of gold as a therapeutic agent for some inflammatory disorders[53]. Cultured murine macrophages were found to withstand the lethal effects of endotoxin (LPS) if they were pretreated with either glucocorticoid or metals that induce MT[59]. Protection was directly related to cellular MT levels. Similarly the natural killer activity of mononuclear cells from patients with AIDS was stimulated when they were incubated with zinc and α-interferon[60]. Both agents induce MT. Zinc ions have many reported actions that may affect the metabolic response of the host to inflammation[61]. It is conceivable that the secretion of IL-1 by macrophages induces hepatic MT production and the transient hypozincaemia that occurs is sufficient to further activate phagocytic cells. Chvapil has proposed that zinc inhibits macrophage migration and phagocytic activity[62].

A key aspect of the cellular function of MT could relate to free radical scavenging activity. A variety of literature suggests that dietary deficiencies of both copper and zinc can lead to lipid peroxidation. Evidence suggests that this effect could be related to depressed superoxide dismutase activity since the cytosolic form of the enzyme contains both metals. However, three independent lines of evidence suggest that MT may act as a free radical scavenger, and in this way prevent deleterious cellular oxidative damage. Purified MT was shown to scavenge both hydroxyl (OH•) and superoxide radicals ($O_2^{-\bullet}$) *in vitro*[63]. Spin trapping studies showed that the rate constant of MT for OH• was 10^6 times greater than for $O_2^{-\bullet}$. Scavenging was accompanied by metal loss and oxidation of thiolate groups, which could be reversed by reduced glutathione and the appropriate metal. It was proposed that MT acts as a renewable protector against OH• mediated oxidations. Since MT is involved in uptake exchange reactions of cells[21], and ligand exchange is rapid[8], this concept is attractive. These observations are supported by other *in vitro* evidence showing an MT-related reduction in lipid peroxidation of erythrocyte membranes[64]. *In vivo* evidence supports this role. Chemically induced lipid peroxidation in isolated rat hepatocytes was induced by a variety of pro-oxidant conditions[30]. Supplementing the culture medium with zinc induced a proportional concentration-dependent increase in MT and decrease in lipid peroxidation. Spin trapping data showed that fewer free radicals were formed in MT-containing hepatocytes.

IV. SUMMARY

Evidence is accumulating that metallothionein has a relationship, perhaps functional in nature, to the inflammatory process. Inducibility of the protein, its characteristic metal-dependent degradation and participation in ligand exchange reactions provide for regulated copper and zinc metabolism at the cellular level. Expression of metallothionein genes is increased by hormones, particularly interleukin-1, that are involved in the response to inflammation. Metallothionein may act as an inducible free radical scavenger to help cells handle the elevated amounts of active oxygen species, particular hydroxyl radicals, produced during inflammation. The involvement of interleukin-1 in the regulation of metallothionein gene expression supports this complex involvement of the protein in inflammation.

Acknowledgement

The authors thank Walter Jones and Dawn Mendoza for preparation of the figure and manuscript, respectively. Research in the laboratory of RJC is supported by the National Institutes of Health and Institute of Food and Agricultural Sciences.

References

1.　　Kagi, JHR and Nordberg, M (eds)(1979). *Metallothionein*. (Basel: Birkhauser Verlag)

2.　　Cousins, RJ (1985). Absorption, transport, and hepatic metabolism of copper and zinc: special reference to metallothionein and ceruloplasmin. *Physiol Rev*, **65**, 238–309

3. Hamer, DH (1986). Metallothionein. *Ann Rev Biochem*, **55**, 913–951
4. Dunn, MA, Blalock, TL and Cousins, RJ (1987). Metallothionein: minireview. *Proc Soc Exp Biol Med*, **185**, 107–119
5. Kagi, JHR and Kokima, Y (eds)(1987). *Metallothionein-2*. (Basel: Birkhauser Verlag), 702 pp
6. Winge, DR and Miklossy, KA (1982). Domain nature of metallothionein. *J Biol Chem*, **257**, 3471–3476
7. Nielson, KB and Winge, DR (1983). Order of metal binding in metallothionein. *J Biol Chem*, **258**, 13063–13069
8. Nettesheim, DG, Engeseth, HR and Otvos, JD (1985). Products of metal exchange reactions of metallothionein. *Biochemistry*, **24**, 6744–6751
9. Nielson, KB, Atkin, CL and Winge, DR (1985). Distinct metal-binding configurations in metallothionein. *J Biol Chem*, **260**, 5342–5350
10. Gurd, FRN and Wilcox, PE (1956). Complex formation between metallic cations and proteins, peptides, and amino acids. In Anson, ML, Bailey, K and Edsall, JT (eds) *Advances in Protein Chemistry*, pp 311–427
11. Durnam, DM and Palmiter, RD (1981). Transcriptional regulation of the mouse metallothionein-I gene by heavy metals. *J Biol Chem*, **256**, 5712–5716
12. Sequin, C and Hamer, DH (1987). Regulation in vitro of metallothionein gene binding factors. *Science*, **235**, 1383–1387
13. Squibb, KS, Cousins, RJ and Feldman, SE (1977). Control of zinc-thionein synthesis in rat liver. *Biochem J*, **164**, 223–228
14. McCormick, CC, Menard, MP and Cousins, RJ (1981). Induction of hepatic metallothionein by feeding zinc to rats of depleted zinc status. *Am J Physiol*, **240**, E414–E421
15. Menard, MP, McCormick, CC and Cousins, RJ (1981). Regulation of intestinal metallothionein biosynthesis in rats by dietary zinc. *J Nutr*, **111**, 1353–1361
16. Blalock, TL, Dunn, MA and Cousins, RJ (1987). Sensitivity of native metallothionein promoters to dietary copper and zinc. *Fed Proc*, **46**, 3313 abs.
17. Oh, SH, Deagan, JT, Whanger, PD and Weswig, PH (1978). Biological function of metallothionein. V. Its induction in rats by various stresses. *Am J Physiol*, **234**, E282–E285
18. Sobocinski, PZ, Canterbury, WJ, Jr, Knutsen, GL and Hauer, EC (1981). Effect of adrenalectomy on cadmium- and turpentine-induced hepatic synthesis of metallothionein and α2-macrofetoprotein in the rat. *Inflammation*, **5**, 153–164
19. Swerdel, MR and Cousins, RJ (1984). Changes in rat liver metallothionein and metallothionein mRNA induced by isopropanol. *Proc Soc Exp Biol Med*, **175**, 522–529
20. Failla, ML and Cousins, RJ (1978). Zinc accumulation and metabolism in primary cultures of rat liver cells: regulation by glucocorticoids. *Biochem Biophys Acta*, **543**, 293–304
21. Pattison, SE and Cousins, RJ (1986). Kinetics of zinc uptake and exchange by primary cultures of rats hepatocytes. *Am J Physiol*, **250**, E677–E685
22. Etzel, KR, Shapiro, SG and Cousins, RJ (1979). Regulation of liver metallothionein and plasma zinc by the glucocorticoid dexamethasone. *Biochem Biophys Res Commun*, **89**, 1120–1126
23. Hager, LJ and Palmiter, RD (1981). Transcriptional regulation of mouse liver metallothionein-I gene by glucocorticoids. *Nature*, **291**, 340–342
24. Karin, M, Haslinger, A, Holtgreve, H *et al.* (1984a). Activation of a heterologous promoter in response to dexamethasone and cadmium by metallothionein gene 5'-flanking DNA. *Cell*, **36**, 371–379
25. Henkin, RI, Foster, DM, Aamodt, RL and Berman, M (1984). Zinc metabolism in adrenalcortical insufficiency: effects of carbohydrate active steroids. *Metabolism*, **33**, 491–501

26. Bremner, I and Davies, NT (1975). The induction of metallothionein in rat liver by zinc injection and restriction of food intake. *Biochem J*, **149**, 733–738
27. Richards, MP and Cousins, RJ (1976). Metallothionein and its relationship to the metabolism of dietary zinc. *J Nutr*, **106**, 1591–1599
28. Cousins, RJ, Dunn, MA, Leinart, AS *et al.* (1986). Coordinate regulation of zinc metabolism and metallothionein gene expression in rats. *Am J Physiol*, **251**, E688–E694
29. Dunn, MA and Cousins, RJ (1987). Regulation of metallothionein gene transcriptional and kinetics of zinc metabolism by dibutyryl cAMP. *Fed Proc*, **46**, 1644 abs.
30. Cousins, RJ and Coppen, DE (1987). Regulation of liver zinc metabolism and metallothionein by cAMP, glucagon and glucocorticoids and suppression of free radicals by zinc. In Kagi, JHR and Kojima, Y (eds) *Metallothionein II*. (Basel: Birkhauser Verlag), pp 545–553
31. Sobocinski, PZ, Canterbury, WJ, Jr, Mapes, CA and Dinterman, RE (1978). Involvement of hepatic metallothionein in hypozincemia associated with bacterial infection. *Am J Physiol*, **234**, E399–E406
32. Feldman, SI and Cousins, RJ (1976). Degradation of hepatic zinc-thionein following parenteral zinc administration. *Biochem J*, **160**, 583–588
33. Etzel, KR, Swerdel, MR, Swerdel, JN and Cousins, RJ (1982). Endotoxin-induced changes in copper and zinc metabolism in the Syrian hamster. *J Nutr*, **112**, 2363–2373
34. Sobocinski, PZ and Canterbury, WJ, Jr (1982). Hepatic metallothionein induction in inflammation. *Ann NY Acad Sci*, **210**, 354–367
35. Durnam, DM, Hoffman, JS, Quaife, CJ *et al.* (1984). Induction of mouse metallothionein-I mRNA by bacterial endotoxin in independent of metals and glucocorticoid hormones. *Proc Natl Acad Sci*, **81**, 1053–1056
36. DiSilvestro, RA and Cousins, RJ (1984). Mediation of endotoxin-induced changes in metabolism in rats. *Am J Physiol*, **247**, E436–E441
37. Klasing, KC (1984). Effect of inflammatory agents and interleukin-1 on iron and zinc metabolism. *Am J Physiol*, **247**, R901–R904
38. Cousins, RJ, Blalock, TL, Barber, EF and Leinart, AS (1987). Regulation of liver metallothionein gene expression by interleukin-1. *Fed Proc*, **46**, 3453 abs.
39. Flynn, A (1983). Effects of antigen stimulation and interleukin-1 on in vivo splenic zinc changes in the A/mouse. *J Am Coll Nutr*, **2**, 205–213
40. Karin, M, Imbra, RJ, Heguy, A and Wong, G (1985). Interleukin-1 regulates human metallothionein gene expression. *Mol Cell Biol*, **5**, 2866–2869
41. Gubler, U, Chua, AO, Stern, AS, Hellmann, CP, *et al.* (1986). Recombinant human interleukin 1α: purification and biological characterization. *J Immunol*, **136**, 2492–2497
42. Klasing, KC, Richards, MP, Darcey, SE and Laurin, DE (1987). Presence of acute phase changes in zinc, iron, and copper metabolism in turkey embryos. *Proc Soc Exp Biol Med*, **184**, 7–13
43. Williams, RJP (1984). Zinc: what is its role in biology? *Endeavor*, **8**, 65–70
44. Weiner, AL and Cousins, RJ (1983). Hormonally produced changes in ceruloplasmin synthesis and secretion in primary cultured rat hepatocytes-relationship to hepatic copper metabolism. *Biochem J*, **212**, 297–304
45. Weiner, AL and Cousins, RJ (1983). Differential regulation of copper and zinc metabolism in rat liver parenchymal cells in primary cultures. *Proc Soc Exp Biol Med*, **173**, 486–494
46. Scheckinger, T, Hartmann, HJ and Weser, U (1986). Copper transport from Cu(I)-thionein into apo-caeruloplasmin mediated by activated leucocytes. *Biochem J*, **240**, 281–283
47. Cousins, RJ and Swerdel, MR (1985). Ceruloplasmin and metallothionein induction by zinc and 13-cis-retinoic acid in rats with adjuvant inflammation. *Proc Soc Exp Biol Med*, **179**, 168–172

48. Willson, RL (1977). Iron, zinc, free radicals and oxygen in tissue disorders and cancer control. In *Iron Metabolism*, pp 331–354. Ciba Foundation Symposium 51 (Amsterdam: Elsevier/Excerpta Medica/North Holland)

49. Halliwell, B and Gutteridge, JMC (1984). Oxygen toxicity, oxygen radicals, transition metals and disease. *Biochem J*, **219**, 1–14

50. Goldstein, IM, Kaplan, HB, Edelseon, HS and Weissman, G (1979). Ceruloplasmin: a scavenger of superoxide anion radicals. *J Biol Chem*, **254**, 4040–4045

51. Milanino, R, Conforti, A, Fracasso, ME, Franco, L, *et al.* (1979). Concerning the role of endogenous copper in the acute inflammatory process. *Agents and Actions*, **9**, 581–588

52. Bakka, A, Endresen, L, Johnsen, ABS, *et al.* (1981). Resistance against cis-dichlorodiammineplatinum in cultured cells with a high content of metallothionein. *Toxicol Appl Pharmacol*, **61**, 215–226

53. Butt, TR, Sternberg, EJ, Mirabelli, CK and Crooke, ST (1985). Regulation of metallothionein gene expression in mammalian cells by gold compounds. *Mol Pharmacol*, **29**, 204–210

54. Bakka, A, Johnsen, AS, Endressen, L and Rugstad, HE (1982). Radioresistance in cells with high content of metallothionein. *Experientia*, (Basel), **38**, 381–383

55. Herrlich,P, Rahmsdor, HJ, Angel, P, Luckehuh, C, *et al.* (1986). Signals and sequences involved in the UV and TPA dependent induction of genes. *J Cell Biol*, (S10C), 108, abs.

56. Shiraishi, N, Yamamoto, H, Takeda, Y, Kondoh, S, *et al.* (1986). Increased metallothionein content in rat liver and kidney following X-irradiation. *Toxicol Appl Pharmacol*, **85**, 128–134

57. Schmitz, G, Minkel, DT, Gingrich, D and Shaw, CF III (1980). The binding of gold(I) to metallothionein. *J Inorg Biochem*, **12**, 293–306

58. Sharma, RP and McQueen, EG (1982). The effect of zinc and copper pretreatment on the binding of gold(I) to hepatic and renal metallothioneins. *Biochem Pharmacol*, **31**, 2153–2159

59. Patierno, SR, Costa, M, Lewis, VM and Peavy, DL (1983). Inhibition of LPS toxicity for macrophages by metallothionein-inducing agents. *J Immunol*, **130**, 1924–1929

60. Cunningham-Rundles, S (1984). Nutritional factors in immune response. In *Malnutrition: Determinants and Consequences*, pp 233–244. (New York: Liss)

61. Mapes, CA, Bailey, PT, Matson, CF, *et al.* (1978). *In vitro* and *in vivo* actions of zinc ion affecting cellular substances which influence host metabolic responses to inflammation. *J Cell Physiol*, **95**, 115–124

62. Chvapil, M (1976). Effect of zinc on cells and biomembranes. *Med Clin N Am*, **60**, 799–812

63. Thornalley, PJ and Vasak, M (1985). Possible role for metallothionein in protection agains radiation-induced oxidative stress. Kinetics and mechanism of its reaction with superoxide and hydroxyl radicals. *Biochim Biophys Acta*, **827**, 36–44

64. Thomas, JP, Bachowski, GJ and Girotti, AW (1986). Inhibition of lipid peroxidation in cell membranes by zinc-metallothione. *Fed Proc*, **45**, 1661, abs.

4

Iron- or copper-dependent lipid peroxidation of lipoproteins at inflammatory sites: potential role in the mediation of tissue damage

JA Cuthbert, PL Jeffrey and PE Lipsky
Liver Unit and Rheumatic Diseases Division
Department of Internal Medicine
The University of Texas Southwestern Medical Center at Dallas
Dallas, Texas, USA

Summary

Oxygen-derived free radicals generated during inflammatory responses contribute to tissue injury by a number of mechanisms including the initiation of lipid peroxidation. This process may directly cause cellular damage or generate toxic intermediates that alter cell function. Rheumatoid arthritis is a chronic inflammatory disease in which the presence and action of free radicals can be examined by studying the contents of the synovial fluid. In rheumatoid synovial fluid there is evidence of lipid peroxidation as indicated by the finding that low-density lipoproteins (LDL) isolated from the fluid contain elevated levels of thiobarbituric acid-reactive substances. Both the mechanism of lipid peroxidation of LDL and the possibility that the altered LDL might contribute to tissue damage were investigated. Similar lipid peroxidation of LDL occurred when plasma LDL was incubated with micromolar concentrations of iron or copper. Peroxidation of LDL was diminished by superoxide dismutase, indicating that the process involved the action of the superoxide anion. The possibility that the altered LDL inhibited cellular function was examined by studying its effect on mitogen-induced lymphocyte proliferation. Marked inhibition of lymphocyte function was noted, that could be correlated with the concentration of thiobarbituric acid-reactive substances in the LDL preparation. The inhibitory effect of the altered LDL was not prevented by superoxide dismutase. The possibility that immunological reactivity might contribute to the peroxidation of LDL was also examined. In these studies a marked increase in copper-dependent superoxide-mediated lipid peroxidation was noted when LDL was incubated with mitogen-

Copper and Zinc in Inflammation. Milanino, R, Rainsford, KD and Velo, GP (eds)
Inflammation and Drug Therapy Series, Volume IV

activated lymphocytes. This finding suggested that lipid peroxidation of synovial fluid LDL may be greatly facilitated by the action of the local immunological activity in the joint space. The results suggest that lipoproteins may have a complex modulatory influence on inflammation. Low levels of LDL may undergo peroxidation, but not to a sufficient degree to become inhibitory of cell function. In this manner LDL may protect other tissues by serving as a terminal 'sink' for free radical reactivity. With more intense inflammation lipid peroxidation of LDL proceeds, causing the altered lipoproteins to become inhibitory of cellular function.

I. INTRODUCTION

Free radical generation is part of many biochemical reactions necessary for normal cell function[1]. Free radicals, however, also have the potential to denature or modify biological molecules[1-4]. In particular, oxygen-derived free radicals, generated during inflammatory responses, have been implicated in the tissue injury associated with acute and chronic inflammation[1,2,4]. One potential mechanism of tissue damage by oxygen-derived free radicals is by the formation of lipid peroxides within cell membranes[1,2,4]. Experimental evidence suggests that lipid peroxidation of membranes leads to structural alterations and abnormal function[1]. In addition, free radicals may alter a variety of normal host constituents, thereby generating peroxy derivatives with inhibitory activity[1-4].

A number of investigators have hypothesized that lipid peroxidation may contribute to the development or progression of inflammatory injury in rheumatoid arthritis[5-8]. Neutrophils, monocytes and tissue macrophages that participate in rheumatoid inflammation are capable of generating oxygen-derived free radicals[1,9]. These inflammatory cells produce the reactive oxygen species superoxide and hydrogen peroxide during the "respiratory burst" that follows activation by phagocytic stimuli or soluble mediators[1,9]. When traces of metal ions such as iron or copper are present, oxygen-derived free radicals may initiate lipid peroxidation[10-14]. In support of this mechanism of tissue injury, Lunec and co-workers have detected lipid peroxidation products in synovial fluid of rheumatoid arthritis patients[5]. Furthermore, Rowley and colleagues have demonstrated that synovial fluid from rheumatoid patients contains thiobarbituric acid-reactive substances (TBARS), indicative of lipid peroxidation, although the specific nature of the oxidized molecules was not identified[8]. The amount of TBARS in rheumatoid synovial fluid correlated with both the concentration of iron in the synovial fluid and with the activity of the inflammatory synovitis[8]. Free radical oxidation products are also significantly elevated in the serum of patients with rheumatoid arthritis, compared to normal controls[6,7]. Moreover, the levels decline after treatment with anti-inflammatory agents, suggesting a correlation with disease activity[7].

The free radical oxidation products in the serum of rheumatoid arthritis patients are associated with lipoproteins[7]. The possibility that synovial fluid lipoproteins may undergo lipid peroxidation and contribute to disease activity has not previously been considered. Synovial fluid normally contains only trace amounts of cholesterol and phospholipid in lipoproteins[15,16]. However, inflammatory processes lead to a marked increase in the concentration of lipoproteins in synovial fluid[16-19]. Levels of low-density lipoprotein (LDL), the most abundant species, are equivalent to 40-60% of normal serum LDL concentrations[16,18,19]. The current studies were undertaken to examine the possibility that lipoproteins in synovial fluid may undergo lipid peroxidation during inflammation and to explore possible mechanisms and consequences of these changes.

II. LIPID PEROXIDATIVE REACTIONS

1. Lipid peroxidation of synovial fluid lipoproteins

In the initial studies, synovial fluid was obtained from patients with rheumatoid arthritis and LDL isolated by sequential ultracentrifugation as described previously[20]. Evidence of lipid peroxidation was detected by measurement of TBARS content and expressed as malondialdehyde (MDA) equivalent content per milligram of lipoprotein cholesterol[21]. As seen in Table 1, there was minimal lipid peroxidation of LDL prepared from normal plasma. In contrast, the TBARS content of synovial fluid LDL was increased by more than 20-fold. This difference is unlikely to result from changes in the lipoproteins occurring during isolation, since EDTA was added to both synovial fluid and plasma before ultracentrifugation. Chelation of trace metals by EDTA has been shown to prevent lipid peroxidation during preparation of lipoproteins[11,12]. Thus, synovial fluid obtained from patients with rheumatoid arthritis contains LDL that has undergone lipid peroxidation *in vivo*.

Table 1 Lipid peroxidation of synovial fluid lipoproteins

LDL	TBARS content* (nmol MDA/mg cholesterol)
Plasma	0.15 ± 0.02
Synovial fluid No.1	3.5
Synovial fluid No.2	6.3

*Lipid peroxidation of low-density lipoprotein (LDL) was measured by quantitating the thiobarbituric acid reactive substances (TBARS) content as described[21]. The data are expressed as malondialdehyde (MDA) equivalent content per milligram of lipoprotein cholesterol. Results are mean of triplicate determinations for synovial fluid and mean ± SEM of nine preparations of plasma LDL.

35

2. Trace metals promote lipid peroxidation of LDL

The next series of experiments examined possible mechanisms of lipid peroxidation of LDL. Trace metals such as iron and copper are known to promote lipid peroxidation[10-14]. Since elevated levels of iron and copper have been detected in rheumatoid synovial fluid[22-24], experiments were carried out to determine whether these could initiate lipid peroxidation of LDL. Plasma LDL was incubated with varying concentrations of iron or copper for 24 h at 37°C and then assayed for TBARS content. As shown in Table 2, incubation of LDL with FeCl3 resulted in lipid peroxidation, as evidenced by a marked increase in TBARS content. Lipid peroxidation was observed with the addition of as little as 10 μM FeCl3 and reached a maximum with 20-25 μM FeCl3. Copper was also able to induce lipid peroxidation of LDL and at high concentrations (> 10 μM) was as effective as iron. These results suggested that lipid peroxidation of LDL may be promoted *in vivo* by trace metal ions such as Cu or Fe in synovial fluid. Of importance, the degree of lipid peroxidation induced *in vitro* by incubation of LDL with iron or copper was comparable to that detected in LDL isolated from rheumatoid synovial fluid.

Table 2 Iron and copper promote lipid peroxidation of LDL

Incubation		TBARS content of LDL* (nmol MDA/mg cholesterol)
Nil		0.0
FeCl3	5 μM	0.0
	10 μM	2.2
	20 μM	29.6
Nil		0.0
CuCl2	0.5 μM	0.0
	5 μM	3.4
	10 μM	6.4

*LDL (200 μg cholesterol/ml) was incubated for 24 h at 37°C with and without varying concentrations of FeCl3 or CuCl2 before measurement of TBARS content. TBARS was measured as described in the legend of Table 1. Results represent mean of triplicate determinations.

3. Iron- and copper-modified LDL inhibits lymphocyte responses

In the next series of experiments the capacity of LDL which had undergone iron-promoted lipid peroxidation to alter cellular function was examined. Since persistent immunological activity is thought to perpetuate rheumatoid inflammation[25], the model of mitogen-induced lymphocyte proliferation was utilized as a means to examine the capacity of altered LDL to affect cellular function. The effect of iron-preincubated LDL on lymphocyte growth was examined initially. Peripheral blood mononuclear cells (PBM) were isolated and cultured as previously described[26]. PBM were stimulated with the mitogenic lectin phytohaemagglutinin (PHA) and the response was measured by assaying lymphocyte DNA synthesis as the incorporation of [3H]thymidine after a 4-day incubation as detailed[20,26]. The addition of control LDL had no effect on lymphocyte DNA synthesis (Table 3). However, when an equal concentration of iron-preincubated LDL was added, responses were completely inhibited. The iron-preincubated LDL had undergone lipid peroxidation, as demonstrated by the elevated TBARS content, suggesting that the inhibitory effect was related to free radical-induced alteration of LDL.

Table 3 Iron-preincubated LDL inhibits lymphocyte responses

Addition to culture	*PHA-induced lymphocyte [3H]thymidine incorporation* * $(cpm \times 10^{-3})$
Nil	206.3 ± 1.9
Control-preincubated LDL	205.5 ± 9.7
FeCl3-preincubated LDL	0.2 ± 0.0

*Peripheral blood mononuclear cells (PBM) were cultured with or without phytohaemagglutinin (PHA) and LDL (100 µg cholesterol/ml) as indicated. Before addition to culture, LDL was preincubated for 24 h at 37°C with or without 100 µM FeCl3. TBARS content was 0.4 nmol MDA/mg cholesterol for control LDL and 10.5 nmol MDA/mg cholesterol for iron-preincubated LDL. Lymphocyte DNA synthesis was measured after 4 days by the incorporation of [3H]thymidine. Unstimulated cultures incorporated <500 cpm. Results are mean ± SEM of triplicate determinations.

The next series of experiments examined whether copper was similar to iron in its capacity to generate an altered LDL and inhibit lymphocyte growth. Preincubation of LDL with 10 µM CuCl2 for 24 h at 37°C resulted in lipid peroxidation (Table 2). When copper-preincubated LDL was added to cultures of mitogen-stimulated PBM, lymphocyte DNA synthesis was inhibited in a manner similar to that caused by iron-preincubated LDL (data not shown). The inhibitory effect was dependent on the concentration of oxidized LDL added, and correlated with the degree of lipid peroxidation as measured by TBARS content.

4. Role of superoxide in the iron-mediated generation of inhibitory LDL

Additional experiments examined the mechanism whereby iron generated an inhibitory LDL. The oxygen-derived free radical superoxide has been shown to initiate lipid peroxidation of LDL in the presence of iron and copper[14].

Table 4 Generation of inhibitory LDL by iron: protection by superoxide dismutase

Addition to culture	PHA-induced lymphocyte [^{3}H]thymidine incorporation* (cpm x 10^{-3})
Nil	181.0 ± 10.1
Control-preincubated LDL	185.5 ± 6.7
Iron-preincubated LDL	9.6 ± 1.1
Iron and SOD-preincubated LDL	89.0 ± 12.1

*Before addition to culture, LDL was preincubated for 24 h at 37°C with saline (control), FeCl3 (100 μM) or FeCl3 and superoxide dismutase (SOD 300 U/ml). After dialysis, the various LDL preparations (40 μg cholesterol/ml) were added to cultures of PHA-stimulated PBM. TBARS content per mg cholesterol were 0.2 nmol MDA (control), 12.6 nmol MDA (iron) and 4.2 nmol MDA (iron and SOD). After 4 days, PHA-induced lymphocyte DNA synthesis was measured by the incorporation of [^{3}H]thymidine. Unstimulated cultures incorporated < 400 cpm. Results are mean ± SEM of triplicate determinations.

Table 5 Inhibition of lymphocyte response by iron-preincubated LDL: lack of protection by superoxide dismutase

LDL added to culture		PHA-induced lymphocyte [^{3}H]thymidine incorporation*	
μg cholesterol/ml	nmol MDA/ml	Medium	SOD
		(cpm x 10^{-3}; percentage inhibition)	
No LDL		176.1 ± 3.3	184.2 ± 13.9
Iron-preincubated			
18	0.2	171.8 ± 3.7 (2%)	187.9 ± 17.1 (0%)
36	0.4	126.3 ± 8.1 (28%)	135.8 ± 12.4 (26%)
54	0.6	8.4 ± 1.6 (95%)	11.4 ± 2.7 (94%)
72	0.8	0.1 ± 0.0 (100%)	0.3 ± 0.1 (100%)
Control-preincubated			
72	0.04	188.7 ± 9.4 (0%)	196.4 ± 13.5 (0%)

*LDL was preincubated for 24 h at 37°C with 100 μM FeCl3, dialysed, and TBARS content of the LDL was determined. Various concentrations of LDL were added to PHA-stimulated cultures in the presence and absence of SOD (300 U/ml). Control LDL was not inhibitory. PHA-induced lymphocyte DNA synthesis was measured after 4 days by the incorporation of [^{3}H]thymidine. Unstimulated cultures incorporated < 300 cpm. Results are mean ± SEM of triplicate determinations.

The role of superoxide in the generation of inhibitory LDL was therefore investigated by using the enzyme superoxide dismutase (SOD) to block its effect. As shown in Table 4, LDL preincubated in saline (control) had no effect on lymphocyte DNA synthesis, whereas LDL preincubated in $FeCl_3$ completely inhibited responses. When LDL was preincubated with iron in the presence of SOD the inhibitory effect was partially abrogated. Inhibition of lymphocyte proliferation by LDL was directly correlated with evidence of lipid peroxidation. Thus, iron pre-incubated LDL had markedly increased TBARS content (12.6 nmol MDA/mg cholesterol) whereas control LDL did not (0.2 nmol MDA/mg cholesterol), and this increase was partially prevented by SOD (4.2 nmol MDA/mg cholesterol for LDL incubated with iron and SOD). These results suggested that superoxide contributed to iron-mediated generation of inhibitory LDL. The role of superoxide in the inhibition of lymphocyte responses by altered LDL was also investigated. For these experiments, iron-preincubated LDL was added to cultures in the presence or absence of SOD. As shown in Table 5, there was a concentration-dependent suppression of mitogen-stimulated DNA synthesis with the addition of iron-preincubated LDL. SOD had no significant effect on the capacity of oxidized LDL to inhibit lymphocyte responses. Therefore, superoxide contributed to the lipid peroxidation of the LDL, but was not involved in the inhibition of cell growth by the altered LDL.

5. Cellular enhancement of lipid peroxidation

It has previously been suggested that lipid peroxidation of LDL in the presence of trace metal ions is increased by the presence of cultured cells that release superoxide[14]. The next series of experiments was undertaken with the aim of exploring the influence of proliferating lymphocytes on copper-dependent lipid peroxidation of LDL and the generation of inhibitory products. The initial experiments utilized PHA-stimulated lymphocytes to examine the inhibitory effects of mixtures of copper and LDL. Neither copper nor LDL alone had any effect on PHA-stimulated lymphocyte DNA synthesis (Table 6). In contrast, when both were added, there was marked inhibition of lymphocyte responses. The addition of LDL (100 μg cholesterol/ml) to cultures containing 0.5 μM $CuCl_2$ resulted in 74% inhibition of PHA-induced lymphocyte DNA synthesis. Inhibition by lower concentrations of LDL also occurred, but required higher concentrations of copper. Of importance, marked LDL-dependent inhibition of responsiveness was noted with concentrations of copper (0.5 μM) that failed to generate lipid peroxidation when incubated with LDL in the absence of PBM (Table 2). These results suggested that the PBM had conferred additional inhibitory effects.

Table 6 Copper-dependent inhibition of lymphocyte responses by LDL

LDL (μg cholesterol/ml)	Copper concentration (μM)			
	Nil	0.05	0.5	5
	PHA-induced lymphocyte DNA synthesis* (cpm x 10⁻³)			
0	145.5 ± 4.4	149.1 ± 12.1	134.3 ± 8.0	149.2 ± 7.5
10	151.0 ± 2.6	138.7 ± 6.2	123.0 ± 4.0	120.0 ± 3.0
50	130.3 ± 2.5	129.2 ± 5.0	120.2 ± 4.8	13.6 ± 2.1
100	158.8 ± 4.3	117.8 ± 5.7	35.1 ± 3.0	0.1 ± 0.0
500	161.1 ± 8.3	102.3 ± 4.2	0.1 ± 0.0	0.1 ± 0.0

*PBM were incubated with or without PHA and varying concentrations of $CuCl_2$ and LDL as indicated. After 4 days PHA-induced lymphocyte DNA synthesis was measured by the incorporation of [³H]thymidine. Unstimulated cultures incorporated < 300 cpm and were unchanged by additions. Results are mean ± SEM of triplicate determinations.

In order to confirm that the generation of inhibitory LDL was enhanced by cellular participation, LDL was preincubated for 24 h at 37°C with varying concentrations of $CuCl_2$ and dialysed before measuring its effect on lymphocyte responses. When added to cultures, neither control-preincubated LDL nor copper-preincubated LDL inhibited mitogen-induced lymphocyte DNA synthesis (Table 7). The lack of an inhibitory effect related to the finding that the degree of lipid peroxidation generated by copper in the absence of cells was insufficient to cause inhibition of lymphocyte growth. Thus, the TBARS content of LDL preincubated with 0.5 and 5.0 μM copper was 0.08 and 0.15 nmol MDA/ml, respectively. The addition of similar concentrations of oxidized LDL generated by iron preincubation (0.2 nmol MDA/ml) likewise did not cause inhibition of lymphocyte responses (Table 5).

Table 7 Preincubation with low concentrations of copper does not generate inhibitory LDL

Addition	Preincubation	PHA-induced lymphocyte [³H]thymidine incorporation* (cpm x 10⁻³)
Nil	–	203.8 ± 3.4
LDL	Control	208.7 ± 3.1
	$CuCl_2$ 0.5 μM	197.1 ± 12.0
	$CuCl_2$ 5.0 μM	219.7 ± 9.0

*LDL was preincubated for 24 h with or without $CuCl_2$ and extensively dialysed before addition to culture. LDL (100 μg cholesterol/ml) was then added to cultures of PHA-stimulated PBM. TBARS content was 0.5 nmol MDA/mg cholesterol for control LDL and 0.8 and 1.5 nmol MDA/mg cholesterol for copper-preincubated LDLs. PHA-induced lymphocyte DNA synthesis was measured after 4 days by the incorporation of [³H]thymidine. Unstimulated cultures incorporated < 400 cpm. Results are mean ± SEM of triplicate determinations.

The role of PBM in promoting lipid peroxidation of LDL by low concentrations of copper was examined in the next experiments. LDL was incubated with PBM and copper for varying lengths of time before the measurement of TBARS content of the LDL-containing supernatant. As shown in Table 8, lipid peroxidation of LDL was increased by incubation with PBM. The greatest effect was observed after 48 h in PHA-stimulated cultures, at which time TBARS content was increased 4-fold and was equivalent to 10 nmol/mg cholesterol. In contrast, preincubation of LDL with copper alone resulted in 0.8-1.5 nmol MDA/mg cholesterol (Table 7). These findings indicated that PHA-stimulated PBM promoted copper-dependent lipid peroxidation of LDL, and that the generation of inhibitory LDL paralleled the degree of lipid peroxidation.

Table 8 Copper-mediated lipid peroxidation: augmentation by PHA-stimulated peripheral blood mononuclear cells

Addition to supernatant	Length of incubation	
PHA-stimulated PBM	24 h	48 h
	Supernatant TBARS content* (nmol MDA/ml)	
Nil	0.2	0.0
Cu^{2+}	0.0	0.1
LDL	0.0	0.4
Cu^{2+} + LDL	0.6	2.0

*PBM were incubated in medium with PHA, $CuCl_2$ (0.5 μM) and LDL (200 μg cholesterol/ml) as indicated. After 24 or 48 h, supernatants were harvested and TBARS content assayed. Results are mean of triplicate determinations.

Table 9 Inhibition of lymphocyte responses by LDL and copper: the role of superoxide

Addition	PHA-induced lymphocyte [³H]thymidine incorporation*			
	Control		LDL	
	Medium	Cu^{2+}	Medium	Cu^{2+}
	cpm x 10⁻³			
Nil	213.3 ± 24.3	158.0 ± 4.8	210.4 ± 6.2	4.8 ± 1.0
SOD	187.9 ± 9.3	144.5 ± 1.6	219.9 ± 10.3	204.9 ± 11.5
Ethanol	142.9 ± 23.1	120.9 ± 10.4	152.5 ± 11.5	4.0 ± 0.2
BHT	128.4 ± 1.0	99.4 ± 6.1	174.2 ± 7.9	135.6 ± 11.3
Nil	121.6 ± 5.1	114.7 ± 4.6	157.6 ± 0.6	0.1 ± 0.0
Catalase	111.8 ± 2.6	99.9 ± 10.0	136.7 ± 7.9	0.1 ± 0.0

*PBM were incubated in medium with or without PHA, $CuCl_2$ (0.5 μM), LDL (200 μg cholesterol/ml) as indicated and with or without BHT (200 μM), SOD (300 U/ml) and catalase (100 U/ml). After 4 days, PHA-induced lymphocyte DNA synthesis was measured by [³H]thymidine incorporation. Unstimulated cultures incorporated < 200 cpm. Results are mean ± SEM of triplicate determinations.

The combination of copper and LDL inhibited lymphocyte responses by a superoxide-dependent mechanism. Thus, superoxide dismutase and butylated hydroxytoluene, a free radical scavenger, completely blocked the suppressive effect (Table 9). In contrast, catalase was ineffective. In summary, the results indicate that copper-dependent superoxide-mediated lipid peroxidation of LDL and the generation of an inhibitory lipoprotein was enhanced by immunologic activity.

III. INFLAMMATION AND LIPID PEROXIDATION OF LIPOPROTEINS

The current studies indicate that lipid peroxidation of synovial fluid lipoproteins occurs during rheumatoid inflammation. LDL isolated from synovial fluid of patients with rheumatoid arthritis had increased levels of TBARS as evidence of lipid peroxidation. In normal synovial fluid there are only trace amounts of lipoproteins[15,16]. With inflammation, however, the permeability of the synovial membrane increases and the lipoprotein concentrations rise[16-19]. Lipoprotein levels in rheumatoid synovial fluid are 10-20-fold elevated when compared with normal synovial fluid, reaching 40-60% of serum levels[16,18,19]. The elevation is not specific for rheumatoid arthritis. Similar increases in synovial fluid lipoproteins have also been observed in osteoarthritis and traumatic arthritis[17,18].

The observation that the lipoproteins in rheumatoid synovial fluid undergo lipid peroxidation suggests that they may play a role in modulating inflammatory responses. Lipid peroxidation is one of the primary mechanisms proposed to explain free radical-mediated cell and tissue injury. Free radicals, produced during inflammation by neutrophils, monocytes and macrophages, initiate lipid peroxidation by interaction with polyunsaturated fatty acids[1,2]. The reaction is propagated by the generation of additional radicals and terminated by the formation of end-products such as MDA and volatile hydrocarbons[1,2]. The formation of lipid peroxides within cell membranes and organelles alters membrane function[1,2]. Moreover, free radicals can be transferred from the lipids to proteins and nucleic acids, causing denaturation and eventual tissue damage[1,2].

Free radical reactions have been implicated in the development of rheumatoid arthritis by a number of investigators[5-8,27-29]. McCord proposed that superoxide produced in an inflamed arthritic joint by activated neutrophils degraded synovial fluid[27]. In addition, superoxide and its metabolites have been shown to denature cartilage proteoglycan and collagen[28]. The current studies indicate that superoxide produced in an inflamed joint causes lipid peroxidation. Each of these free radical reactions may contribute to the disease process.

Evidence of lipid peroxidation in rheumatoid arthritis has been demonstrated by other investigators[5-8]. Lunec and co-workers found fluorescent degradation products of free radical oxidation in synovial fluid and serum, but were unable to detect thiobituric acid-reactive compounds[5]. However, Rowley and colleagues were able to detect thiobarbituric acid-reactive material in serum and synovial fluid of rheumatoid patients[8]. The current studies clearly indicate that the lipid peroxidation products previously identified in synovial fluid were lipoproteins.

1. Role of iron

The mechanism of lipid peroxidation of synovial fluid LDL remains speculative. However, the present experiments demonstrate that either copper or iron can cause lipid peroxidation of LDL by a mechanism involving superoxide. Blake and colleagues have proposed that iron which accumulates in rheumatoid synovial membrane and fluid contributes to the inflammatory process by promoting lipid peroxidation[30]. The iron in synovial fluid is stored predominantly as ferritin[24]. In rheumatoid arthritis the synovial ferritin may be 20 times the corresponding serum value[24]. Protein-bound iron may be unable to catalyse lipid peroxidation[31]. However, superoxide derived from stimulated neutrophils is able to mobilize iron from ferritin[32]. Furthermore, unlike other forms of protein-bound iron, ferritin has been shown to stimulate lipid peroxidation[33]. Since there are superoxide-producing cells and iron mobilized from ferritin in synovial fluid during inflammation, the conditions are suitable for lipid peroxidation of synovial fluid LDL.

Iron may also cause lipid peroxidation by a mechanism that is independent of superoxide. Thus, SOD only partially abrogated the effect of preincubation of LDL with iron (see Section II(4)). Similar results have been reported by Heinecke and colleagues[14]. They found that lipid peroxidation of LDL incubated with smooth muscle cells was dependent on the addition of trace metals[13,14]. SOD diminished but did not completely prevent lipid peroxidation catalysed by iron, whereas copper-mediated lipid peroxidation was entirely blocked by SOD[14]. There are a number of other mechanisms to account for iron-mediated superoxide-independent lipid peroxidation[2,10,30]. Thus, iron could directly promote lipid peroxidation by reacting with performed lipid hydroperoxides[10]. The current studies suggest that such lipid hydroperoxides may be present in plasma LDL, as indicated by the small but detectable amount of thiobarbituric acid-reactive material in plasma LDL immediately following isolation. Stable lipid hydroperoxides can become reactive in the presence of iron and initiate further lipid peroxidation[10]. Such a mechanism may account for iron-generated superoxide-independent lipid peroxidation of LDL. Alternatively, iron may react with hydroxyl radicals to initiate lipid peroxidation[2,30]. Like superoxide, hydroxyl radicals are products of stimulated phagocytes[9]. Although iron catalyses hydroxyl radical formation from the combination of superoxide and hydrogen peroxide, it can also catalyse hydroxyl radical formation directly from hydrogen peroxide[1,2,10]. Once formed, the highly reactive hydroxyl radicals are able to initiate lipid peroxidation[1,2,10]. Therefore, iron-mediated lipid peroxidation independent of superoxide may result from reactivity with preformed lipid hydroperoxides or as the consequence of hydroxyl radical formation. Either of these mechanisms may contribute to lipid peroxidation in synovial fluid.

2. Copper-dependent reactions

Alternatively, synovial fluid LDL may be oxidised by superoxide in a copper-dependent mechanism. Of note, very low concentrations of copper generated inhibitory LDL in the presence of immunological activity. Patients with rheumatoid arthritis have elevated levels of copper in serum and synovial fluid which may promote lipid peroxidation[22,34-36]. Although most of the elevated copper is associated with caeruloplasmin, elevated urinary copper values suggest that non-protein-bound copper may also be abnormally high in rheumatoid arthritis[35]. The current studies demonstrate that non-protein-bound copper is able to promote superoxide-mediated lipid peroxidation of LDL in agreement with other investigators[13,14]. The capacity of copper in caeruloplasmin to substitute for non-protein-bound copper in this system has not been determined. Caeruloplasmin copper is able to replace free copper in the generation of reactive oxygen species that modulate lymphocyte function in other systems[37]. Thus, Lipsky has shown that D-penicillamine and other thiols markedly suppressed lymphocyte function when copper ions were present[37]. Copper complexes and caeruloplasmin were also able to inhibit lymphocyte responses when added with D-penicillamine[37]. The effect of D-penicillamine and copper on lymphocyte responses was somewhat different from that described in the current report, since hydrogen peroxide was the toxic species although superoxide was an intermediary. In other systems, caeruloplasmin has been shown to protect against lipid peroxidation[38]. Therefore copper may be active in catalysing lipid peroxidation of synovial fluid LDL in rheumatoid arthritis; alternatively, iron or both metal ions may be responsible for promoting the free radical reaction.

3. Effects of oxidized LDL

Oxidized LDL, once generated, may contribute to disease progression. LDL that has undergone lipid peroxidation has been shown to be cytotoxic for a number of different cultured cells, including lymphocytes, fibroblasts and vascular cells[11,39,40]. Synovial cells may be similarly affected. In the current studies the altered LDL suppressed proliferation of cultured lymphocytes. Large numbers of lymphocytes are present in rheumatoid synovial fluid and tissue, suggesting they play an important role in the chronic inflammation that is a hallmark of rheumatoid arthritis. Prevention of lymphocyte proliferation by the altered LDL may modulate this inflammatory response. Soluble mediators and cytokines released by proliferating lymphocytes may contribute to the resolution of the inflammatory response and be important in repair mechanisms[41]. Suppression of lymphocyte proliferation by altered LDL may therefore exacerbate chronic inflammation by interfering with production of these factors.

The current studies indicate that superoxide is no longer involved once the inhibitory LDL has been generated. In addition, the inhibition of lymphocyte function by iron-preincubated LDL is not prevented by other free radical scavengers. Thus, altered LDL has the capacity to continue to cause cell damage after the lipid peroxidation reaction has terminated. Alternatively, the altered LDL may act as an intermediate in the free radical reactions and contribute to the denaturation of other structures. Lunec and colleagues[29] have detected the evidence of free radical reactions involving synovial fluid immunoglobulin G. They were able to produce similar changes in immunoglobulin G with peroxidized arachidonic acid[29]. Arachidonic acid is found in the phospholipid fraction of LDL and is likely to be peroxidized by free radical reactions. Immunoglobulin G altered by peroxidizing lipid may then stimulate additional superoxide generation with subsequent tissue damage[29]. Therefore, lipid peroxidation of LDL may serve as a marker and indicate the presence of other oxygen-derived free radical damage.

Finally, the possibility that lipid peroxidation of LDL may have beneficial effects cannot be completely excluded. Oxidation of LDL may result in termination of a lipid peroxidation reaction by formation of malondialdehyde and other conjugates, without denaturation or damage of other structures. If the lipid peroxidation reaction was terminated when the content of thiobarbituric acid-reactive material was low, the current studies suggest that there would be no deleterious effect. Oxidized LDL could therefore be protective by absorbing oxygen radicals and effectively terminating lipid peroxidation. Tissue damage would not be expected if the concentration of altered LDL remained low. Alternatively, if high concentrations of oxidized LDL are generated they might suppress inflammatory responses and modulate disease activity by inhibiting lymphocyte function. Treatment of rheumatoid arthritis by modalities that inhibit lymphocyte proliferation can lead to remission of disease activity[37,42-45]. Thus, D-penicillamine is an effective anti-inflammatory agent in rheumatoid arthritis and may act by inhibiting lymphocyte responses[36]. In addition, cytotoxic drugs and other therapies that inhibit cell proliferation are efficacious in the treatment of rheumatoid arthritis[42-45]. Inhibition of lymphocyte proliferation by oxidized LDL may also be beneficial in a similar manner. The correlation of lipid peroxidation products with disease activity renders this alternative less likely[7]. However, a small or incomplete beneficial effect may be masked in the setting of severe disease.

IV. CONCLUSIONS

In conclusion lipid peroxidation of LDL occurs in synovial fluid in rheumatoid arthritis. Potential mechanisms resulting in lipid peroxidation of LDL include reactions dependent on superoxide and micromolar concentrations of iron and/or copper. Moreover, lipid peroxidation of LDL is likely to be facilitated by the action of a number of cell types participating in the chronic inflammation. LDL that has undergone lipid peroxidation inhibits cell growth as evidenced by suppression of mitogen-stimulated lymphocyte responses. Oxidized LDL may contribute to the pathogenesis of rheumatoid arthritis by inhibiting cell function or by transferring free radical activity to other target molecules.

Acknowledgements

This work was supported in part by grants AI7653 and AM09989 from the National Institutes of Health.

References

1. Fantone, JC and Ward, PA (1982). Role of oxygen-derived free radicals and metabolites in leukocyte-dependent inflammatory reactions. *Am J Pathol*, **107**, 397-418
2. Halliwell, B and Gutteridge, JMC (1984). Oxygen toxicity, oxygen radicals, transition metals and disease. *Biochem J*, 219, 1-14
3. McCord, JM (1985). Oxygen-derived free radicals in postischemic tissue injury. *N Engl J Med*, 312, 159-163
4. Halliwell, B and Gutteridge, JMC (1984). Lipid peroxidation, oxygen radicals, cell damage, and antioxidant therapy. *Lancet*, 1, 1396-1397
5. Lunec, J and Dormandy, TL (1979). Fluorescent lipid-peroxidation products in synovial fluid. *Clin Sci*, 56, 53-59
6. Muus, P, Bonta, IL and den Oudsten, SA (1979). Plasma levels of malondialdehyde, a product of cyclo-oxygenase-dependent and independent lipid peroxidation in rheumatoid arthritis: a correlation with disease activity. *Prostagland Med*, 2, 63-65
7. Lunec, J, Halloran, SP, White, AG and Dormandy, TL (1981). Free-radical oxidation (peroxidation) products in serum and synovial fluid in rheumatoid arthritis. *J Rheumatol*, 8, 233-245
8. Rowley, D, Gutteridge, JMC, Blake, D *et al.* (1984). Lipid peroxidation in rheumatoid arthritis: thiobarbituric acid-reactive material and catalytic iron salts in synovial fluid from rheumatoid patients. *Clin Sci*, 66, 691-695
9. Babior, BM (1984). The respiratory burst of phagocytes. *J Clin Invest*, 73, 599-601
10. Aust, SD and Svingen, BA (1982). The role of iron in enzymatic lipid peroxidation. *Free Radicals in Biology*, V, 1-28
11. Morel, DW, Hessler, JR and Chisolm, GM (1983). Low density lipoprotein cytotoxicity induced by free radical peroxidation of lipid. *J Lipid Res*, 24, 1070-1076
12. Steinbrecher, UP, Parthasarathy, S, Leake, DS *et al.* (1984). Modification of low density lipoprotein by endothelial cells involves lipid peroxidation and degradation of low density lipoprotein phospholipids. *Proc Natl Acad Sci, USA*, 81, 3883-3887
13. Heinecke, JW, Rosen, H and Chait, A (1984). Iron and copper promote modification of low density lipoprotein by human arterial smooth muscle cells in culture. *J Clin Invest*, 74, 1890-1894
14. Heinecke, JW, Baker, L, Rosen, H and Chait, A (1986). Superoxide-mediated modification of low density lipoprotein by arterial smooth muscle cells. *J Clin Invest*, 77, 757-761
15. Schmid, K and MacNair, MB (1958). Characterization of the proteins of certain postmortem human synovial fluids. *J Clin Invest*, 37, 708-718
16. Bole, GG (1962). Synovial fluid lipids in normal individuals and patients with rheumatoid arthritis. *Arthritis Rheum*, 5, 589-601
17. Schmid, K and MacNair, MB (1956). Characterization of the proteins of human synovial fluid in certain disease states. *J Clin Invest*, 35, 814-824
18. Small, DM, Cohen, AS and Schmid, K (1964). Lipoproteins of synovial fluid as studied by analytical ultracentrifugation. *J Clin Invest*, 43, 2070-2079

19. Viikari, J, Jalava, S and Terho, T (1980). Synovial fluid lipids in rheumatoid arthritis. *Scand J Rheum*, 9, 164-166
20. Cuthbert, JA and Lipsky, PE (1983). Immunoregulation by low density lipoproteins in man: Low density lipoprotein inhibits mitogen-stimulated human lymphocyte proliferation after initial activation. *J Lipid Res*, 24, 1512-1524
21. Buege, JA and Aust, SD (1978). In Sleischer, F and Packer, L (eds) *Methods in Enzymology*, vol.52, pp.302-310. (New York: Academic Press)
22. Scudder, PR, McMurray, W, White, AG and Dormandy, TL (1978). Synovial fluid copper and related variables in rheumatoid and degenerative arthritis. *Ann Rheum Dis*, 37, 71-72
23. White, AG, Scudder, P, Dormandy, TL and Martin, VM (1978). Copper - an index of erosive activity. *Rheum Rehabil*, 17, 3-5
24. Blake, DR, Bacon, PA, Eastham, EJ and Brigham, K (1980). Synovial fluid ferritin in rheumatoid arthritis. *Br Med J*, 281, 715-716
25. Zvaifler, NJ (1973). The immunopathology of joint inflammation in rheumatoid arthritis. *Adv Immunol*, 16, 265-336
26. Cuthbert, JA and Lipsky, PE (1986). Promotion of human T lymphocyte activation and proliferation by low density and high density lipoproteins. *J Biol Chem*, 261, 3620-3627
27. McCord, JM (1974). Free radicals and inflammation: protection of synovial fluid by superoxide dismutase. *Science*, 185, 529-531
28. Greenwald, RA and May, WW (1979). Inhibition of collagen gelation by action of superoxide radical. *Arthritis Rheum*, 22, 251-259
29. Lunec, J, Blake, DR, McCleary, SJ *et al.* (1985). Self-perpetuating mechanisms of immunoglobulin G aggregation in rheumatoid inflammation. *J Clin Invest*, 76, 2084-2090
30. Blake, DR, Hall, ND, Bacon, PA *et al.* (1981). The importance of iron in rheumatoid disease. *Lancet*, 2, 1142-1144
31. Baldwin, DA, Jenny, ER and Aisen, P (1984). The effect of human serum transferrin and milk lactoferrin on hydroxyl radical formation from superoxide and hydrogen peroxide. *J Biol Chem*, 259, 13391-13394
32. Biemond, P, van Eijk, HG, Swaak, AJG and Koster, JF (1984). Iron mobilization from ferritin by superoxide derived from stimulated polymorphonuclear leukocytes. Possible mechanism in inflammation disease. *J Clin Invest*, 73, 1576-1579
33. Gutteridge, JMC, Halliwell, B, Treffry, A *et al.* (1983). Effect of ferritin-containing fractions with different iron loading on lipid peroxidation. *Biochem J*, 209, 557-560
34. Scudder, PR, Al-Timimi, D, McMurray, W *et al* (1978). Serum copper and related variables in rheumatoid arthritis. *Ann Rheum Dis*, 37, 67-70
35. Aaseth, J, Munthe, E, Forre, O and Steinnes, E (1978). Trace elements in serum and urine of patients with rheumatoid arthritis. *Scand J Rheum*, 7, 237-240
36. Brown, DH, Buchanan, WW, El-Ghobarey, AF *et al.* (1979). Serum copper and its relationship to clinical symptoms in rheumatoid arthritis. *Ann Rheum Dis*, 38, 174-176
37. Lipsky, PE (1984). Immunosuppression by D-penicillamine in vitro. Inhibition of human T lymphocyte proliferation by copper- or ceruloplasmin-dependent generation of hydrogen peroxide and protection by monocytes. *J Clin Invest*, 73, 53-65
38. Biemond, P, Swaak, AJG and Koster, JF (1984). Protective factors against oxygen free radicals and hydrogen peroxide in rheumatoid arthritis synovial fluid. *Arthritis Rheum*, 27, 760-765
39. Schuh, J, Fairclough, GF, Jr and Haschemeyer, RH (1978). Oxygen-mediated heterogeneity of apo-low-density lipoprotein. *Proc Natl Acad Sci USA*, 75, 3173-3177
40. Evensen, SA, Galdal, KS and Nilsen, E (1983). LDL-induced cytotoxicity and its inhibition by anti-oxidant treatment in cultured human endothelial cells and fibroblasts. *Atherosclerosis*, 49, 23-30

41. Larsen, GL and Henson, PM (1983). Mediators of inflammation. *Ann Rev Immunol*, 1, 335-359

42. Paulus, HE, Machleder, HI, Levine, S *et al.* (1977). Lymphocyte involvement in rheumatoid arthritis: studies during thoracic duct drainage. *Arthritis Rheum*, 20, 1249-1262

43. Kotzin, BL, Strober, S, Engleman, EG *et al.* (1981). Treatment of intractable rheumatoid arthritis with total lymphoid irradiation. *N Engl J Med*, 305, 969-976

44. Trentham, DE, Belli, JA, Anderson, RJ *et al.* (1981). Clinical and immunologic effects of fractionated total lymphoid irradiation in refractory rheumatoid arthritis. *N Engl J Med*, 305, 976-982

45. Cooperating Clinics Committee of the American Rheumatism Association (1970). A controlled trial of cyclophosphamide in rheumatoid arthritis. *N Engl J Med*, 283, 883-889

5

Copper therapy of inflammatory disorders in man: special reference to rheumatoid arthritis

Felix Fernandez-Madrid
Department of Internal Medicine
Wayne State University School of Medicine
Gordon Scott Hall of Basic Sciences
Detroit, MI 48201, USA

I. INTRODUCTORY HISTORY

There is a resurgence of interest in the essential metals, particularly copper and zinc, in the treatment of the rheumatic diseases.

Mankind has been fascinated with the 'healing' properties of copper for thousands of years. Copper bracelets were known in Mesopotamia and Egypt and were worn by patients in ancient Greece seeking relief of arthritis several thousands of years ago. Even in those times, the mines of Cyprus supplied the metal in such large amounts that the island, Kypros itself, gave its name to copper[1].

Recently, serious attempts have been made to test the possible effects of the copper bracelet on the rheumatic diseases. It has been shown that metallic copper may dissolve in sweat and can be absorbed through the skin[2]. Penetration of copper through the skin was demonstrated in cats, pigs, cattle and humans. Walker *et al.* showed that milligram amounts of copper disappeared after wearing the bracelet[2,3]. These interesting studies clearly showed that metallic copper can be absorbed through the skin and can contribute to increase body copper in a person wearing a bracelet. Wearers of copper bracelets for a period of one month reported less severe degrees of suffering than non wearers and previous users of the bracelet were significantly worse when not wearing their copper bracelets. As to the clinical usefulness of the copper bracelet in rheumatoid arthritis the issue remains unproven since the diagnosis of the population of patients studied was uncertain and rheumatoid arthritis was probably not well represented in the sample[4]. Although little is known about the fate and the possible action of dissolved copper absorbed through the skin, it has recently been shown in animal models of in-

Copper and Zinc in Inflammation. Milanino, R, Rainsford, KD and Velo, GP (eds)
Inflammation and Drug Therapy Series, Volume IV

flammation that dissolved copper from implants possesses anti-inflammatory activity[5].

II. COPPER AND ITS COMPLEXES IN RHEUMATOID ARTHRITIS

In 1940 German investigators began to use organic copper compounds in the treatment of tuberculosis[6], and this work was followed by that of Fenz who used the copper complex Cupralene, sodium-meta-(allylcuprothiocarbamido)-benzoate to treat rheumatoid arthritis[7]. At that time it was thought that rheumatoid arthritis was probably an infectious process and patients with this disease were examined in the trials of the effects of heavy metals. This sequence of events was similar to the first reports of the use of gold for the treatment of rheumatoid arthritis by Lande in 1927, following earlier reports of the beneficial effects of this heavy metal in the treatment of tuberculosis[8]. Forestier, who greatly stimulated the interest in chrysotherapy with his report in 1929[9], also used organic copper compounds in the treatment of rheumatoid arthritis[10]. Forestier and Certonciny treated 50 patients with various types of arthritis, two-thirds of whom may have had rheumatoid arthritis[11]. Their results using Cupralene, which contained 19% of copper, were similar in efficacy to those previously reported using gold salts[9] and largely comparable to those of Fenz[7]. Forestier *et al.* also used Dicuprene, diethylamine-(cupro-oxyquinoline)-sulphonate, another copper complex containing 6.5% copper, and reported that this treatment acted quicker and more effectively than gold in relatively early cases of rheumatoid arthritis[12-15]. Forestier used copper salts in chronic cases of rheumatoid arthritis when gold failed or produced side-effects, and found that the tolerance of copper therapy was superior to that of gold salts. Conflicting data were reported by Kuzell *et al.*[16], who evaluated Dicuprene and Cupralene in patients with rheumatoid arthritis and other rheumatic diseases. These authors reported that only 19.5% of treated patients improved, fewer than those previously observed by Short and Bauer to improve with simple supportive therapy[17]. Thus, Kuzell *et al.* could not confirm the beneficial effects of copper previously reported in rheumatoid arthritis[7,10-15]. Later clinical studies reported that Hangarter and Lubke[18] partially supported the results of Fenz, and Forestier *et al.* Toxicity from copper therapy was reported to be minimal in the studies of Fenz[7], and Forestier *et al.*[10-15], as well as in those of Hangarter *et al.*[18,19] and Kuzell *et al.*[16]. Local pain was noted with the intramuscular injections of Dicuprene, which could be avoided by adding a local anaesthetic. When Cupralene escaped from the vein, pain and local necrosis followed. Hangarter administered Permalon, a copper salicylate preparation by i.v. route to more than 1000 patients with a variety of diagnoses including rheumatic fever, rheumatoid arthritis and sciatica. Rapid relief of symptoms was reported, and 65% of these patients became symptom-free after treatment[19]. Hangarter concluded that the effect of Permalon was not due to salicylate alone, since much higher doses of the latter were needed to achieve therapeutic improvement.

Although the methods used in these early studies[7,10-16,18,19] reflected the state of the art at that time, their evaluation has proven difficult because of problems in the experimental design related to the selection and clinical evaluation of the patients, the diagnostic criteria used, and the lack of controls. In spite of these shortcomings and, in particular, the absence of controlled observations, the fact remains that treatment of a number of patients with rheumatoid arthritis with organic copper salts produced at that time promising results and did merit further investigation. However, while controlled studies subsequently established the beneficial effect of gold for rheumatoid arthritis, treatment with copper became extinct. The decline in the experimental use of parenteral copper in the treatment of rheumatoid arthritis coincided with the surge of corticosteroids and later with the extensive use of non-steroidal anti-inflammatory drugs. The history of the use of copper salts in the rheumatic diseases has been reviewed in detail by Sorenson and Hangarter, who reported on the outcome of about 1500 patients with various rheumatic disorders treated with copper complexes[20].

III. ACTIONS OF COPPER IN INFLAMMATORY CONDITIONS

In spite of the fact that copper complexes have not been used directly in the treatment of rheumatoid arthritis for several decades, with the exception of the experimental use of superoxide dismutase, there are good reasons for discussing how copper is involved in some forms of therapy presently used, and why treatment with copper complexes is potentially a viable therapeutic alternative for the future.

Copper is now recognized as an essential metalloelement[21]. Ionic copper has high affinity for certain ligands, and thus all measurable copper in biological systems exists as complexes or chelates composed of copper bonded to organic components of these systems[22]. In the past four decades considerable experimental work has shown that changes in levels of circulating copper are consistently found in physiological and pathological conditions. The early discovery that serum copper rises during pregnancy[23] was amply confirmed by subsequent studies[24]. The main reason for the rise of serum copper in pregnancy is an elevation of the ceruloplasmin level[25]. Pregnancy-associated remissions, as well as postpartum relapses, are common in patients with rheumatoid arthritis[26]. The effect of pregnancy on the activity of rheumatoid arthritis has been tentatively attributed to the temporal effect of a fetal graft of suppressor cells[27]. However, Denko has proposed that this effect of pregnancy is the result of the protective anti-inflammatory action of increased serum ceruloplasmin[28]. Small doses of estrogens were reported to result in dramatic elevation in serum copper[29] and significantly higher levels of serum copper have been reported in women taking oral contraceptives than in controls[30]. In this context, it is of interest that epidemiological studies have suggested that the intake of oral contraceptives may prevent the development of rheumatoid arthritis[31], although the results of this study need confirmation.

(1) Ceruloplasmin

It is well known that an elevated serum copper level is a feature of numerous inflammatory conditions in animals and man[32-47]. Indeed, data show that circulatory levels of copper rise significantly during the course of acute and chronic inflammatory processes including rheumatoid arthritis. Large quantities of copper complexes appear as part of acute-phase reactants in inflammatory conditions, resulting in an increase in blood copper complex concentrations. The major portion of copper in plasma is tightly bound to ceruloplasmin[48]. This metalloprotein, which contains six to eight atoms of tightly bound copper, accounts for up to 95% of the total copper concentration in blood. It is of interest that increased plasma copper, almost entirely in the form of ceruloplasmin, appears to be an intrinsic response to inflammation[28,48]. This consistent elevation of ceruloplasmin level found in inflammation suggests the intriguing possibility that the enzyme participates in the host defence mechanism. Denko[28], Laroche et al.[48], and Scudder et al.[40] have reported data supporting the anti-inflammatory role of ceruloplasmin. Milanino et al. suggested that copper, copper-zinc superoxide dismutase (SOD), ceruloplasmin and low molecular weight copper chelates may act as scavengers of free radicals, chiefly superoxide anions produced in vivo by activated phagocytes. The scavenging action on free radicals may modulate the overall inflammatory process. Some of the contradictory findings reported on the copper status of patients with rheumatoid arthritis[49] may be explained in part by differences in disease activity, concomitant drug administration or nutritional status. Although ceruloplasmin-bound copper accounts for most of the elevation of serum copper levels in patients with rheumatoid arthritis, non-ceruloplasmin-bound copper also seems to be elevated[35,36,38]. A large body of experimental work supports the view that endogenous copper has an anti-inflammatory activity, and that the elevation of serum copper and ceruloplasmin concentrations observed in acute and chronic inflammatory disease, both in man and animals, has a modulatory role on inflammation as a part of the anti-inflammatory response of the organism[28,33,40,50,51]. The extensive literature on the role of copper in inflammation has recently been reviewed[33,47,52-54].

(2) Superoxide scavenging

In the past two decades considerable evidence has established the importance of free radicals as mediators of the inflammatory response[55]. It was recognized that the superoxide radical ($O_2^{-\bullet}$), can be produced in biological reactions[56,57]. McCord showed that enzymatically generated superoxide radical can depolymerize purified hyaluronic acid and bovine synovial fluid[57]. Since phagocytosing polymorphonuclear leukocytes produce superoxide radical, this reaction was shown to be quantitative feasible as one of the *in vivo* mechanisms of synovial fluid degradation in an inflamed joint[57]. Products of lipid peroxidation have been demonstrated in the synovial fluid of patients with rheumatoid arthritis, indicating a local action of free oxygen radicals[58]. It was proposed that the superoxide radical is an important agent of the toxicity of oxygen and that the enzyme superoxide dismutase constitutes the primary defence against this radical[56,57,59]. Copper and zinc are components of the enzyme superoxide dismutase which detoxifies oxygen. The superoxide dismutases are a group of metalloproteins whose function appears to protect cells against the toxic effects of endogenously generated superoxide radicals[59]. The enzymatic activity of superoxide dismutase was described in 1969 by McCord and Fridovich[60], but its anti-inflammatory activity had been discovered empirically earlier[61]. Rheumatoid arthritis has been associated with decreased copper-zinc SOD activity in polymorphonuclear leucocytes[62,63] and erythrocytes[64]. These studies give support to the experimental use of superoxide dismutase and drugs with SOD-like activity in the treatment of rheumatoid arthritis and other rheumatic disorders[65-68].

Orgotein, the SOD preparation tested in human disease, can reduce inflammation when injected intra-articularly. This protein has been reported to be effective in controlling joint swelling in rheumatoid arthritis[69]. SOD is the only copper-containing drug currently used experimentally in man. The anti-inflammatory properties of Orgotein have been evaluated in animals and man[69], and the safety of this enzyme has been demonstrated by acute, subacute and chronic toxicological studies[70]. The enzyme, which is a relatively large molecule with a molecular weight of 32,000 daltons, has a short half-life of 0.5 hours when injected intravenously in man. Injected Orgotein is rapidly distributed throughout the body but is not taken up by cells. The half-life of SOD injected intra-articularly is presumably longer, but it has not been determined. Furthermore, its protein nature does not permit its oral administration, since the enzyme is susceptible to proteolysis in the gastrointestinal tract. The possibility that the antigenicity of the enzyme may eventually lead to loss of efficacy or to hypersensitivity reactions has not been a major problem in previous work with SOD[70], but long-term observations in humans have not been reported. This is important because osteoarthritis and rheumatoid arthritis are chronic diseases which frequently require a life-long treatment. For these reasons it is unlikely that the present type of SOD will become a major therapeutic alternative in the treatment of the rheumatic diseases in the future. However, the discovery of the involvement of superoxide radicals in inflammation[55,57,58] and the role of superoxide dismutase[59,60] have opened an attractive field of investigation.

It is clear that the use of small molecular weight copper chelates could theoretically be more advantageous than that of superoxide dismutase. It is known that a number of amino acid-copper complexes can act as free-radical scavengers, and it has been established that hydrated copper ions and copper chelated by amino acids or bound to superoxide dismutase or ceruloplasmin have the ability to catalyse the dismutation of superoxide radicals[71]. Copper chelates of some drugs and of amino acids have a small molecular weight, are lipophilic and can rapidly enter cells. It has been reported that many antirheumatic drugs are free radical scavengers or inhibitors of free radical generation[53].

Generation of free radicals is associated with inflammation at multiple levels. They are produced by activated polymorphonuclear leucocytes[72], and as a side product of prostaglandin biosynthesis[73]. Oxygen-derived free radicals can increase vascular permeability *in vivo*[74], produce chemotatic factors[75] and trigger the arachidonic acid cascade[76] which contributes to produce more free radicals as by-products of prostaglandin biosynthesis. Finally, free radicals may produce cellular damage causing the release of lysosomal enzymes and endogenous antigens[34]. Free radicals may be generated by radiation, enzymatic reactions or by the interaction of copper and iron with reducing substances in the presence of oxygen. Prevention of lipid peroxidation can be accomplished by decreasing the accessibility of free radicals to lipids, or by the use of free radical scavengers, which react with free radicals and render them less harmful.

(3) Ambivalence of copper in inflammation

The ambivalent role of copper in inflammatory disorders has been actively investigated and discussed[77]. In addition to the extensive literature supporting the anti-inflammatory role of copper there are reports implicating copper as a destructive agent[38,78]. Whitehouse suggested that drugs, nutritional factors and the disease process can affect the movement of copper between inert, pharmacoactive and toxic forms[77]. It has been proposed that Cu^{2+} and H_2O_2 may contribute to the destruction of cartilage proteoglycan and collagen in inflammatory joint diseases[79]. It is known that free uncomplexed iron and copper ions are toxic, being able to catalyse the formation of hydroxyl radicals[80]. Although copper has the capacity of generating free radicals, paradoxically it can effectively be involved in the scavenging of superoxide radicals in biological systems. Some labile Cu(II) complexes such as Cu(II) bisglycinate are irritant, and can have proinflammatory effects, but copper thiol complexes often have an anti-inflammatory action[81]. It has been shown that copper is a potent inhibitor of bone resorption *in vitro*[82,83]. The stimulation of bone resorption by exogenous prostaglandins was decreased, and the inhibition of bone resorption seen with indomethacin was increased, in the presence of Cu^{2+}. The action of Cu^{2+} in inhibiting bone resorption *in vitro* appears complex but does not involve inhibition of prostaglandin synthesis[82,83].

Bonta showed that copper compounds have anti-inflammatory effects in animals[84], and Sorenson confirmed and extended these findings[52,54,81]. As indicated by Milanino *et al.*[33], copper is active *per se* as an anti-inflammatory agent regardless of the chemical form in which it is administered inorganic copper[85], copper complexes with simple organic molecules with or without anti-inflammatory properties of their own[51,52], copper atoms bound to SOD or SOD-like molecules[56,60] and metallic copper implants[5]. The anti-inflammatory effect of copper complexes can, at least in part, be explained as suggested by Bonta et al.[86]. During phagocytosis, superoxide radicals are released by neutrophils[87] and are also produced by the pathway of prostaglandin biosynthesis[88]. If these free radicals are not scavenged by the inadequate scavenging mechanisms normally present in the body (levels of superoxide dismutase in the extracellular fluid are very low), they will react with biologically important molecules, denaturing proteins and proteoglycans and reacting with membrane fatty acids, resulting in lipid peroxidation[88]. Inhibition of superoxide-mediated lipid peroxidation at the inflamed site leads to a decrease in chemotactic substances and proteolytic enzymes from granulocytes and macrophages. This may explain some of the anti-inflammatory effects of copper chelates which are effective superoxide scavengers.

Sorenson considered the possibility that salicylates, other NSAIDs and some slow-acting drugs commonly utilized in the treatment of rheumatoid arthritis, such as D-penicillamine, owe part of their pharmacological activity to interactions with metal ions and with copper in particular[81]. He demonstrated that copper chelates of low molecular weight have potent anti-inflammatory properties, and discussed various possible mechanisms of action for copper complexes in inflammation[51,52]. Certain metal ions such as Cu^{2+} and Zn^{2+} are known to affect linioleic acid metabolism[89], and are thereby capable of altering the biosynthesis of prostaglandins, for which linoleic acid metabolites are essential precursors. Metal ions are also likely to be involved in several dioxygenase reactions, and might therefore be expected to influence the synthesis of prostaglandins from arachidonic acid and other similar substrates[90]. Sorenson reported that some copper complexes of anti-arthritic drugs have more potent anti-inflammatory effect than the parent drugs in experimental models of inflammation[81], and proposed the interesting hypothesis that the active metabolites of the anti-arthritic drugs are their copper complexes. Other studies have subsequently only in part confirmed the increased potency of the copper complexes over the parent compounds in experimental models of inflammation[91-94]. The rationale behind these apparently contradictory results has been ably discussed by Lewis[91] and by Lewis et al.[85]. The anti-inflammatory effects of copper compounds are dependent on the structure and stability of the complex, the species and the model of inflammation used for testing, the route of administration, as well as the vehicle. If we discount the examples of gastric inactivation and the counterirritation phenomenon[94], there are still a number of copper complexes which appear to possess anti-inflammatory actions[94,95]. It is known that D-penicillamine reduces the free copper fraction in the serum, and that copper-D-penicillamine complexes have SOD-like activity[96]. Penicillamine, like several other thiols, can form mixed disulphides with sulphur-containing proteins. Through these reactions, D-penicillamine can protect thiol groups against the attack of free radicals[97]. Formation of mixed disulphides can also be involved in liberation of protein-bound glutathione within cells, and in making the glutathione peroxidase/reductase system more effective[98].

The interesting proposal that endogenous levels of trace metals can be at the basis of the mechanism of action of slow-acting drugs in the treatment of rheumatoid arthritis deserves further investigation[33]. Clinical studies in patients with rheumatoid arthritis have demonstrated a reduction of the previously elevated levels of serum copper after corticosteroid, gold sodium thiomalate and D-penicillamine therapy[40]. Although results contradictory to this were reported by Smith *et al.*[99], other studies have indicated that therapeutic agents can induce changes in uptake or organ distribution of trace metals. Thus Niedermeier *et al.* reported that injectable gold salts induce a redistribution of trace elements in the body, and can reduce serum concentration of other metals such as tin, molybdenum, manganese, barium and caesium, but not copper, iron or zinc[42]. Thus, except for penicillamine, the ability of the major slow-acting drugs used in the treatment of rheumatoid arthritis to interfere with copper metabolism is controversial[40,95,99,100]. It is likely that studies describing the overall copper status of patients with rheumatoid arthritis, including the identification of low molecular weight copper complexes present in the non-ceruloplasmin fraction of the serum, ceruloplasmin, and total amount of copper contained in the liver and synovial tissue, could help to answer this question.

IV. COPPER MANIPULATION STRATEGIES

Since copper is a metalloelement essential for the function of endogenous superoxide dismutase and ceruloplasmin, the potential role of these enzymes in prevention of tissue damage and in the host defence mechanism is intriguing. Milanino *et al.*[33] suggested two plausible therapeutic strategies in the treatment of chronic inflammatory disorders: the administration of exogenous copper and the *in vivo* manipulation of endogenous metal levels. These principles cannot be immediately applied to the treatment of rheumatoid arthritis because our knowledge of the copper status in this disease is still inadequate. A functional copper deficiency has been assumed but not demonstrated in chronic inflammatory disease[81,101]. Sorenson has suggested that a marginal nutritional deficiency of copper may exist in humans, leading to impaired function of copper-dependent enzymes critical for the host defense mechanism. The studies of Milanino *et al.*[34,46], and that of Denko[28] performed in animals, strongly suggest that copper deficiency is an aggravating factor of inflammation, and support the hypothesis that endogenous copper may play a protective role in inflammation. In the particular case of rheumatoid arthritis, one could ask the question whether a marginal copper deficiency could be a factor leading to chronicity of the inflammatory reaction. In this vein, Rainsford has proposed that marginal copper deficiency, possibly due to dietary and/or environmentally induced changes in the levels of certain trace metals which influence the copper status, may be contributing factors in the pathogenesis of rheumatoid arthritis[101]. Since it has been traditional to assume that measurement of copper in plasma can be used to assess copper nutrition, the elevated values of copper found in patients with rheumatoid arthritis may indicate that the requirements for copper are met in this condition. However, it has been pointed out that in the presence of chronic inflammation the determination of plasma copper has little value in the nutritional assessment of this trace element[102]. It has also been shown that tissue depletion of copper can occur when plasma values are normal[103]. Balance studies performed in the past 40 years have suggested the adult requirement of copper of 2 mg/day[104], and it has been assumed that the average American diet provides more than adequate copper for copper balance[105]. However, there are reports suggesting that daily dietary intake less than 2 mg of copper can occur in the United States[103,106-108], and from previous surveys it appears that the intake of zinc and copper in the US is below the recommended levels[106]. However, since there are no reports of balance studies of copper in patients with rheumatoid arthritis, the question whether marginal copper deficiency is a feature of this disease remains to be answered.

(1) D-Penicillamine

Renewed interest in the role of copper in the treatment of rheumatoid arthritis was stirred by a series of observations on the effect of D-penicillamine on macroglobulins and rheumatoid factors[109,110]. A number of D-penicillamine copper complexes, including Cu(I), Cu(II) and mixed valency states, have been described, and it has been proposed that the formation of a stable copper-D-penicillamine complex that possesses SOD activity is associated with the antirheumatic action of the drug[111]. Interest in the possible effect of copper in the treatment of rheumatoid arthritis was further stimulated by the report of Lipsky and Ziff that D-penicillamine and copper salts have a synergistic inhibitory effect on human lymphocyte proliferation[112]. Several studies had previously suggested that D-penicillamine may have some effect on immune responsiveness[113-117]. Although animal studies did not show a consistent immunosuppressive action of D-penicillamine[118-121], clinical trials[122,123] had previously demonstrated that treatment with this drug does have a beneficial effect on the course of rheumatoid arthritis. Although the administration of penicillamine is known to produce a variety of interesting effects at the biochemical levels, such as the prevention of collagent cross-linking[124], deaggregation of macroglobulins including rheumatoid factor[109,110], inhibition of DNA synthesis[125] and interference with polymorphonuclear leucocyte chemotaxis[126], the mechanism underlying its therapeutic effect is not clearly related to any of the above-mentioned effects of the drug. Most hypotheses attempting to explain the activity of D-penicillamine in the treatment of rheumatoid arthritis assume that the active moieties are the free thiol form of the drug or a copper-penicillamine complex. D-penicillamine is known to form complexes with various metal ions including copper[127]. Whitehouse *et al.*[128] and Sorenson[52] have suggested that copper-penicillamine complexes are the active moieties underlying the effect of D-penicillamine treatment of RA. These authors proposed that penicillamine may sequester copper *in vivo*, and that the circulating low molecular weight complexes formed between copper and penicillamine may contribute to the overall action of the drug. Whitehouse *et al.* further suggested a dual action of penicillamine in transforming inert (protein-bound) copper into pharmacoactive copper and Cu(II), which has the potential to promote inflammation, into innocuous copper[128].

As discussed above, Sorenson proposed that copper coordination compounds may be responsible for the anti-inflammatory activity of antiarthritic preparations[52]. Although this hypothesis has not received sufficient experimental support with the exception of D-penicillamine, Sorenson found that while the parent compound is inactive in test models of inflammation even at large screening doses, two copper coordination compounds obtained with D-penicillamine were found to be active[52].

The mechanism of action of D-penicillamine in Wilson's disease is clearly related to its ability to chelate and mobilize copper[129], but the mechanism of action of the drug in rheumatoid arthritis is not clear. D-penicillamine is a trifunctional amino acid able to participate in oxidation-reduction reactions, sulphydryl-disulphide interchange, and nucleophilic additions, as well as metal binding[130]. Lengfelder *et al.* have shown that copper-penicillamine complexes are able to catalyse the dismutation of superoxide radical[131]. Muijsers *et al.* have reported that copper-penicillamine complexes can be formed *in vivo* during the treatment of patients with rheumatoid arthritis with D-penicillamine leading to measurable plasma SOD activity[132]. In agreement with data previously reported[117,120,133], the studies of Lipsky and Ziff[112] indicated that D-penicillamine alone has a modest inhibitory effect on mitogen-induced human lymphocyte proliferation. However, the inhibition of mitogen responsiveness was markedly augmented by adding copper salts to the culture medium containing D-penicillamine[112]. In those experiments no other divalent cation (zinc, iron, mercury or gold) could produce the increase of the inhibition of mitogen responsiveness observed when copper was added to the cultures along with D-penicillamine. Other thiols which have been shown to be potentially effective in the treatment of rheumatoid arthritis[134-136] could also mediate the copper-dependent inhibition of mitogen responsiveness. Lipsky and Ziff suggested that a complex was formed in culture between the thiol and the copper ion, and that this D-penicillamine-copper complex is the inhibitory moiety[112,137].

A number of observations support the idea that humoral as well as cell-mediated immune processes play an essential role in the maintenance and chronicity of rheumatoid inflammation[138-140]. It has been suggested that agents such as D-penicillamine, which can influence the activity of rheumatoid arthritis, may be active because of their ability to modulate the persistent immune response that characterizes the chronic inflammatory process[112,137]. Data presented by Lipsky and Ziff suggested that penicillamine-copper complexes interfere with the functional ability of T lymphocytes, supporting the possibility that this drug selectively inhibits T cell function through a complex with copper[141]. The inhibition of T cell responsiveness was induced by concentration of both D-penicillamine and copper that might well be expected to be found in patients treated with D-penicillamine[141].

A feature common to all slow-acting drugs used in the treatment of rheumatoid arthritis is that only 50-70% of all patients will respond to the drug. The rest of the patients develop adverse effects, or do not benefit from the drug, for unknown reasons[140]. Muijsers *et al.* reported that serum D-penicillamine levels were the same for patients who responded well to treatment and for those who did not respond. Measurement of penicillamine in serum is complicated by the presence of metabolic products such as penicillamine disulphide, mixed disulphides with both cysteine and protein thiol groups, and S-methyl penicillamine[142]. Muijsers *et al.*[132] reported that half of the D-penicillamine excreted in the urine of rheumatoid arthritis patients is in the form of cysteine-penicillamine mixed disulphide, in agreement with the report of Perrett *et al.*[142]. They observed a marked decrease in the total serum cysteine plus cystine concentration[132]. Munthe *et al.* have found that some non-responders to D-penicillamine treatment could be converted to responders by supplementation with L-cysteine[98].

Another interesting phenomenon which is common to all disease-modifying drugs utilized in the treatment of rheumatoid arthritis is the secondary therapeutic failure after an initial success. It has been reported that administration of D-penicillamine decreases the serum copper levels in patients with rheumatoid arthritis[40,100], supporting the possibility that a relative copper deficiency induced by the increased excretion of copper may be instrumental in the secondary failure of the drug. Dormandy suggested that perhaps the initial effect of the drug is due to the chelate of copper-penicillamine, and once the mobilizable copper in the body has been exhausted the drug ceases to be effective. He suggested that copper supplementation in those patients may prolong the beneficial effect of penicillamine[143]. Osterberg[144] studied Cu(I) complexes of penicillamine in a model system for the *in vivo* reaction between penicillamine and copper (I). This study showed that penicillamine interacts with Cu(I) ions *in vivo*, and that within a certain concentration range the therapeutic use of penicillamine will not disturb the normal Cu(I) metabolism. However, in view of the work of Lipsky and Ziff[112,137,141], it is likely that copper may be the limiting factor prevening the formation of the active complexes. Balance studies of copper and zinc in patients with rheumatoid arthritis treated with D-penicillamine, as well as characterization of penicillamine–copper complexes, could help to discover why some patients with rheumatoid arthritis fail to respond to penicillamine or experience a reactivation after an initial response. Mery *et al.* have reported that even the modest zinc supplementation of 5 mg of zinc per day inhibits the clinical efficacy of D-penicillamine in the treatment of rheumatoid arthritis[145]. The mechanism by which administration of zinc abrogates the effect of D-penicillamine is not known, but it is probably not related to the antagonistic effect of high levels of dietary zinc on copper absorption and status[146]. However, it is of interest that even the ingestion of moderately high amounts of zinc (50 mg/day) which are readily available over-the-counter in pharmacies and food stores, has been shown to decrease the copper status as assessed by erythrocyte Cu, Zn superoxide dismutase[147].

V. SUMMARY AND CONCLUSIONS

In summary, the role of copper in the treatment of rheumatoid arthritis deserves further investigation. Basic questions to be answered relate to the distribution of copper in the tissues and the involvement of copper in the different compartments of the body, including liver and synovial tissue from patients with rheumatoid arthritis before and after the activity of the disease has been modified by the use of slow-acting drugs. Such studies could show whether manipulation of endogenous copper levels in patients with rheumatoid arthritis is a viable therapeutic alternative. Balance studies of copper and zinc in patients with rheumatoid arthritis and appropriate controls should answer the question whether a marginal copper deficiency is a feature of rheumatoid arthritis. If this is proven to be the case, carefully controlled studies involving dietary or dermal supplementation could be of interest. The interesting work on SOD has opened a new and fascinating field of research in the treatment of rheumatic diseases, and the search for small molecular weight copper complexes with superoxide dismutase activity can in the future lead to major advances in therapy. The identification of low molecular weight complexes present in the non-ceruloplasmin bound fraction of sera from patients with rheumatoid arthritis and from normal sera can further our understanding of the protective role of copper in inflammation. The anti-inflammatory action of some copper complexes, and the discovery of the effects of D-penicillamine-copper complexes on the immune system, suggest that pursuing these lines of investigation can lead to an understanding of the modulatory action of copper in chronic inflammation.

References

1. Neuberger, M (1910). *History of Medicine*. (London: Bedford Medical Publications)
2. Walker, WR and Keats, DM (1976). An investigation of the therapeutic value of the copper bracelet. Dermal assimilation of copper in arthritic/rheumatoid conditions. *Agents Actions*, **6**, 454-9
3. Walker, WR (1982). The results of a copper bracelet clinical trial and subsequent studies. In: Sorenson, JRJ (ed), *Inflammatory Diseases and Copper*, (Clifton, NJ: Humana Press) pp. 469-78

4.   Simkin, P. In: Sorenson, JRJ (ed), *Inflammatory Diseases and Copper*, (Clifton, NJ: Humana Press), pp.

5.   Dollwet, HH, Schmidt, SP and Seaman, RE (1981). Antiinflammatory properties of copper implants in the rat paw edema: a preliminary study. *Agents Actions*, **11**(6/7), 746-9

6.   Goralewski, G (1940). Das Kupfer in der Behandlung der lungentuberkulose. *Z Tuberk*, **84**, 313-19

7.   Fenz, E (1941). Kupfer ein neues Mittel gegen chronischen und subacuten Gelenk-rheumatismus. *Münch Med Wochenchschr*, **88**, 1101-5

8.   Lande, K (1927). Die günstige Beeinflussung schleichender Dauerinfecte durch Solganal. *Münch Med Wochenschr*, 74, 1132-4

9.   Forestier, JM (1929). L'aurothérapie dans les Rhumatismes Chroniques. *Bull Mem Soc Med Hop Paris*, 53, 323-7

10.   Forestier, J (1946). Indications et technique des composés organo-metalliques de cuivre dans le Rhumatisme chronique. *Bull Acad Med Paris*, 130, 298-9

11.   Forestier, JM and Certonciny, A (1946). Le Treatment des rhumatismes chroniques par les sels organiques de cuivre. *Presse Med*, 54, 884-5

12.   Forestier, JM, Jacqueline, F and Lenoir, S (1948). La Cuprothérapie intramusculaire dans les rhumatismes chroniques inflammatoires. *Presse Med*, 56, 351-2

13.   Forestier, JM (1949). Comparative results of copper salts and gold salts in rheumatoid arthritis. *Ann Rheum Dis*, **8**, 132-4

14.   Forestier, JM and Certonciny, A (1949). La goutte polyarticulaire chronique et son traitment par les metaux lourds. *Bull Acad Med*, 133, 243

15.   Forestier, JM, Certonciny, A and Jacqueline, F (1950). Therapeutic value of copper salts in rheumatoid arthritis. *Stanford Med Bull*, **8**, 12-13

16.   Kuzell, WC, Schaffarzick, RW, Markle, EA and Gardner, GM (1951). Copper treatment of experimental and clinical arthritis. *Ann Rheum Dis*, **10**, 328-36

17.   Short, CL and Bauer, W (1948). Course of rheumatoid arthritis in patients receiving simple medical and orthopaedic measures. *N Engl J Med*, **238**, 142-8

18.   Hangarter, W and Lubke, A (1952). Über die behandlung rheumatischer erkrankungen mit einer kuper natrium salicylate-complex verbindung. Permalon. *Dtsch Wochenschr*, 77, 870-2

19.   Hangarter, W (1974). *Die salicylsaure und ihre Abkommlinge-Ursprung, Wirkung und Anwendung in der Medizine.* (New York; FK Schattauer Verlag), pp. 312-15

20.   Sorenson, JR and Hangarter, W (1977). Treatment of rheumatoid and degenerative diseases with copper complexes: a review with emphasis on copper-salicylate. *Inflammation*, **2**, 217-38

21.   Underwood, EJ (1977). *Trace Elements in Human and Animal Nutrition*, 4th edn. (New York: Academic Press), pp. 56-108

22.   Sorenson, JRJ (1978). An evaluation of altered copper, iron, magnesium, manganese and zinc concentrations in rheumatoid arthritis. *Inorg Perspect Biol Med*, **2**, 1-26

23.   Krebs, HA (1928). Über das Kupfer in menschlichen blutserum. *Klin Wochenschr*, **7**, 584-5

24.   Thomson, RHS and Watson, D (1949). Serum copper levels in pregnancy and preeclampsia. *J Clin Pathol*, **2**, 193-6

25.   Lahey, ME, Gobler, CJ, Cartwright, GE and Wintrobe, MM (1953). Studies on copper metabolism - VII Blood copper in pregnancy and various pathological states. *J Clin Invest*, **32**, 329-39

26.   Persellin, RH (1976). The effects of pregnancy on rheumatoid arthritis. *Bull Rheum Dis*, **27**, 922-7

27.   Froelich, CJ, Goodwin, JS, Banhurst, A and Williams, RC (1980). Pregnancy: a temporal fetal graft of suppressor cells in autoimmune disease. *Am J Med*, **69**, 329-31

28.   Denko, CW (1979). Protective role of ceruloplasmin in inflammation. *Agents and Actions*, **9**, 333-6

29. Russ, EM and Raymunt, J (1956). Influence of estrogens in total serum copper and ceruloplasmin. *Proc Soc Exp Biol Med*, **92**, 466-6

30. Crews, MG, Taper, LJ and Ritchey, SJ (1980). Effects of oral contraceptive agents on copper and zinc balance in young women. *Am J Clin Nutr*, **33**, 1940-5

31. Royal College of General Practitioners (1974). *Oral Contraceptive Study: oral contraceptives and health*. (London: Pitman Medical Publishing)

32. Van Ravesteijn, S (1945). Over de Koperstofwisseling by den mensch en over het kopergehalte van het blet by normale en zieke personen. MD Thesis. Utrecht. P Den Boer

33. Milanino, R, Conforti, A, Franco, L *et al*. (1985). Review: Copper and inflammation – a possible rationale for the pharmacological manipulation of inflammatory disorders. *Agents and Actions*, **16**, 504-13

34. Milanino, R and Velo, GP (1981). Multiple actions of copper in control of inflammation: studies in copper-deficient rats. In: Rainsford, KD, Brune, K and Whitehouse, MW (eds), *Trace Elements in the Pathogenesis and Treatment of Inflammation*. (Basel: Birkhauser Verlag), pp. 209-30

35. Niedermeier, W (1969). Concentration and clinical state of copper in synovial fluid and blood serum of patients with rheumatoid arthritis. *Ann Rheum Dis*, **24**, 544-8

36. Grennan, DM, Knudson, JM, Dunckley, J *et al*. (1980). Serum copper and zinc in rheumatoid arthritis and osteoarthritis. *NZ Med J*, **91**, 47-50

37. Plantim, IO and Strandberg, PO (1965). Whole-blood concentrations of copper and zinc in rheumatoid arthritis studied by activation analysis. *Acta Rheum Scand*, **11**, 30-4

38. Lorber, A, Cutler, LS and Chang, CC (1968). Serum copper levels in rheumatoid arthritis: relationship of elevated copper to protein alterations. *Arthr Rheum*, **11**, 65-71

39. Sorenson, JRJ and DiTommaso, D (1976). Significance of plasma copper and caeruloplasmin concentrations in rheumatoid arthritis. *Ann Rheum Dis*, **35**, 186-8

40. Scudder, PR, Al-Timini, D, McMurray, W *et al*. (1978). Serum copper and related variables in rheumatoid arthritis. *Ann Rheum Dis*, **37**, 67-70

41. Niedermeier, W, Creitz, EE and Holley, HL (1962). Trace metal composition of synovial fluid from patients with rheumatoid arthritis. *Arth Rheum*, **5**, 439-444

42. Niedermeier, W, Prillman, WM and Griggs, JH (1971). The effect of chrysotherapy on trace elements in patients with rheumatoid arthritis. *Arth Rheum*, **14**, 533-8

43. Conforti, A, Franco, L, Milanino, R *et al*. (1982). Copper and ceruloplasmin activity in rheumatoid arthritis. In: Gorkin, S, Ziff, M, Velo, GP and Gorini, S (eds), *Advances in Inflammation Research*, Vol.3: *Rheumatoid Arthritis*. (New York: Raven Press), pp. 237-44

44. Koj, A (1970). Acute-phase reactants and lysosomal enzymes in the blood of rats with experimental inflammation or radiation injury. *Fol Biol*, **18**, 274-86

45. Wintrobe, MM, Cartwright, GE and Gubler, CJ (1953). Studies on the function and metabolism of copper. *J Nutr*, **50**, 395-419

46. Milanino, R, Mazzoli, S, Passarella, E *et al*. (1978). Carrageenan edema in copper-deficient rats. *Agents Actions*, **8**, 618-22

47. Milanino, R, Conforti, A, Fracasso, ME *et al*. (1979). Concerning the role of endogenous copper in the acute inflammatory process. *Agents and Actions*, **9**, 581-8

48. Laroche, MJ, Chappuis, P, Henry, Y and Rousselet, F (1982). Ceruloplasmin. Experimental anti-inflammatory activity and physicochemical properties. In: Sorenson, JBL (ed), *Inflammatory Diseases and Copper*. (Clifton, NJ: Humana Press), pp. 61-74

49. Bajpayee, DP (1975). Significance of plasma copper and ceruloplasmin concentrations in rheumatoid arthritis. *Ann Rheum Dis*, **34**, 162-7

50. Milanino, R, Passarella, E and Velo, GP (1979). Copper and the inflammatory pro-

cess. In: Weismann, G *et al.* (eds), *Advances in Inflammatory Research*, Vol.I. (New York: Raven Press), pp. 281-91

51. Sorenson, JRJ (1977). Evaluation of copper complexes as potential antiarthritic drugs. *J Pharm Pharmacol*, 29, 450-2

52. Sorenson, JRJ (1976). Copper chelates as possible active forms of the antiarthritic agents. *J Med Chem*, 19, 135-48

53. Bonta, I, Parnham, MJ, Vincent, JE and Bragt, PC (1980). In: Ellis, PG and West GB (eds), *Progress in Medicine and Chemistry*. (Amsterdam: Elsevier/North Holland), vol.17, pp. 185-273

54. Sorenson, JRJ (1981). In: Rainsford, KD *et al.* (eds), *Trace Elements in the Pathogenesis and Treatment of Inflammation*. (Basel: Basel Birkhauser Verlag), p.305

55. Salin, ML and McCord, JM (1975). Free radicals and inflammation. Protection of phagocytosing leukocytes by superoxide dismutase. *J Clin Invest*, 56, 1319-23

56. McCord, JM and Fridovich, I (1968). The reduction of cytochrome c by milk xantine oxidase. *J Biol Chem*, 243, 5753-60

57. McCord, JM (1974). Free radicals and inflammation. Protection of synovial fluid by superoxide dismutase (SOD). *Science*, 185, 529-31

58. Lunec, J, Halloran, SP, White, AG and Dormandy, TL (1981). Free radical oxidation (peroxidation) products in serum and synovial fluid in rheumatoid arthritis. *J Rheumatol*, 8, 233-45

59. Fridovich, I (1975). Superoxide dismutase. *Ann Rev Biochem*, 44, 147-59

60. McCord, JM and Fridovich, I (1969). Superoxide dismutase: an enzymic function for erythrocuprein (hemocuprein). *J Biol Chem*, 244, 6049-55

61. Huber, W, Schulte, TL, Carson, S *et al.* (1968). Some chemical and pharmacological properties of a novel anti-inflammatory protein. *Toxicol Appl Pharmacol*, 12, 308

62. Rister, M, Bauermeister, K, Gravert, V and Gladtke, E (1978). Superoxide dismutase deficiency in rheumatoid arthritis. *Lancet*, 1(8073), 1094

63. Pasquier, C, Laoussadi, S, Serfati, G *et al.* (1985). Superoxide dismutases in polymorphonuclear leukocytes from patients with ankylosing spondylitis or rheumatoid arthritis. *Clin Exp Rheum*, 3, 123-6

64. Banford, JC, Brown, DH, Hazelton, RA *et al.* (1982). Serum copper and erythrocyte superoxide dismutase in rheumatoid arthritis. *Ann Rheum Dis*, 41, 458-62

65. Lund-Olespm, K and Menander, KB (1974). Orgotein: A new anti-inflammatory metalloprotein drug: Preliminary evaluation of clinical efficacy and safety in degenerative joint disease. *Curr Therap Res*, 16, 706-17

66. Puhl, W, Biehl, G, Kelgel, R and Hefer, M (1981). *Eur J Rheumatol Inflamm*, 4, 264

67. Huskisson, EC and Scott, J (1981). Orgotein in osteoarthritis of the knee joint. *Eur J Rheumatol Inflamm*, 4, 212-8

68. Wolf, B (1982). Therapy of inflammatory diseases with superoxide dismutase. In: Sorenson, JRJ (ed), *Inflammatory Diseases and Copper*. (Clifton, NJ: Humana Press), pp. 453-670

69. Huber, W, Menander-Huber, KB, Saifer, MGP and Dang, PHC (1977). Studies on the clinical and laboratory pharmacology of drug formulations of bovine Cu-Zn superoxide dismutase (Orgotein). In: Willoughby, DA *et al.* (eds), *Perspectives in Inflammation*. (Lancaster: MTP Press), pp. 527-44

70. Carson, S, Vagin, EE, Huber, W and Schulte, TL (1973). Safety tests of orgotein, an anti-inflammatory protein. *Toxicol Appl Pharmacol*, 26, 184-202

71. Bonta, IL, Bragt, PC and Muus, P (1982). Hepatic adaptation process during inflammatory conditions. Role of trace elements, lipid peroxidation and ceruloplasmin. In: Sorenson, JRJ (ed), *Inflammatory Diseases and Copper*. (Clifton, NJ: Humana Press), pp. 243-53

72. Fridovich, I, McCord, JM and Michelson, AM (1977). Epilogue and prospects. In: Michelson, AM *et al.* (eds), *Superoxide and Superoxide Dismutase*. (New York: Academic Press), pp. 551-6

73. Kuehl, FA, Jr, Humes, JL, Egan, RW et al. (1977). Role of prostaglandin endoperoxide PGG$_2$ in inflammatory processes. Nature, 256, 170-3

74. Biork, J, Del Maestro, RF and Arfos, KE (1980). Evidence for participation of hydroxyl free radicals in increase microvascular permeability. In: Velo, GP (ed), Trends in Inflammation Research, Vol.I. (Basel: Birkhauser Verlag), pp. 208-13

75. McCord, JM, Stokes, SM and Wong, K (1979). Superoxide radicals as a phagocyte-producer chemical mediator of inflammation. In: Weissman, G (ed), Advances in Inflammation Research, Vol.I. (New York: Raven Press), pp. 273-80

76. Oyanagui, Y (1976). Participation of superoxide anions in the prostaglandin phase of carrageenan foot-oedema. Biochem Pharmacol, 25, 1465-72

77. Whitehouse, Y (1976). Ambivalent role of copper in inflammatory disorders. Agents and Actions, 6, 201-6

78. Gerber, A (1974). Copper catalized thermal aggregation of human gamma globulin. Arthr Rheum, 17, 85-91

79. Chung, MH, Kesner, L and Chan, PC (1984). Degradation of articular cartilage by copper and hydrogen peroxide. Agents and Actions, 15(3/4), 328-35

80. Blake, RD, Hall, ND, Bacon, PA et al. (1981). The importance of iron in rheumatoid disease. Lancet, 2, 1142-4

81. Sorenson, JRJ (1982). Copper complexes as the active metabolites of anti-inflammatory agents. In: Sorenson, JRJ (ed), Inflammatory Disease and Copper. (Clifton, NJ: Humana Press), pp. 289-301

82. Wilson, T, Katz, JM and Gray, DH (1981). Inhibition of active bone resorption by copper. Calcif Tissue Int, 33, 35-9

83. Katz, JM, Skinner, SJM, Wilson, T and Gray, DH (1984). Inhidbition of prostaglandin action and bone resorption by copper. Ann Rheum Dis, 43, 841-6

84. Bonta, IL (1969). Microvascular lesions as a target of anti-inflammatory and certain other drugs. Acta Physiol Pharmacol Neerl, 15, 188-222

85. Lewis, AJ, Cattney, J, Teape, J et al. (1978). Copper and its involvement in the inflammatory process. Eur J Rjeumatol Inflamm, 1, 295-9

86. Bonta, IL, Bragt, PC and Muus, P (1982). Hepatic adaptation process during inflammatory conditions. Role of trace elements, lipid peroxidation and ceruloplasmin. In: Sorenson, JRJ (ed), Inflammatory Disease and Copper. (Clifton, NJ: Humana Press), pp. 243-53

87. Babier, BM, Kipnes, RS and Carnutte, A (1973). Biological defence mechanisms: the production by leukocytes of superoxide. J Clin Invest, 52, 741-4

88. Bragt, PG, Schenkelaars, EPM and Bonta, IL (1979). Dissociation between prostaglandin and malonyldialdehyde formation in exudate and measured levels of malonyldialdehyde in plasma and liver during granulation inflammation in the rat. Prostaglandins Med, 2, 51-61

89. Cunnane, SC (1981). Zinc and copper interact antagonistically in the regulation of linolenic acid metabolism. Prog Lipid Res, 20, 601-3

90. Nugteren, DH, Beerthuis, RK and van Dorp, DA (1966). The enzymic conversion of all-cis-8,11,14-eicosatrienoic acid into prostaglandin E$_1$. Rec Trav Chim, 85, 405

91. Boyle, E, Freeman, PC, Goudie, AC et al. (1976). The role of copper preventing gastrointestinal damage by acidic anti-inflammatory drugs. J Pharm Pharmacol, 28, 865-8

92. Williams, DA, Walz, DT and Foye, WO (1976). Synthesis and biological evaluation of Tetrakis (acetylsalicylate)-u-dicopper (II). J Pharm Sci, 65, 126-8

93. Rainsford, KD and Whitehouse, MW (1976). Concerning the merits of copper aspirin as a potential anti-inflammatory drug. J Pharm Pharmacol, 28, 83-6

94. Lewis, AJ (1984). The role of copper in inflammatory disease. Agents and Actions, 15, 511-19

95. Lewis, AJ, Smith, WE and Brown, DH (1981). A comparison of the anti-inflammatory activities of copper complexes in different models of inflammation. In: Rains-

ford, KD *et al.* (eds), *Trace Elements in the Pathogenesis and Treatment of Inflammation. Agents and Actions* Suppl. Vol.8. (Basel: Birkhauser Verlag), pp.

96. Langfelder, E and Elsever, EF (1978). Determination of the superoxide dismutating activity of D-penicillamine copper. Hopper Seylers Zeitschr. *Physiol Chem*, **359**, 51-757

97. Munthe, E, Aaseth, J and Jellum, E (1986). Trace elements and rheumatoid arthritis (RA). Pathogenetic and therapeutic aspects. *Acta Pharmacol Toxicol*, **59**, 365-73

98. Munthe, E, Koss, E and Jellum, E (1981). D-penicillamine-induced increase in intracellular glutathione correlating to clinical response in rheumatoid arthritis. *J Rheumatol*, **8**, 14-19

99. Smith, WE, Brown, DH, Dunlop, J *et al.* (1980). The effect of therapeutic agents on serum copper levels and serum oxidase activities in the rat adjuvant model compared to analogous results from studies of rheumatoid arthritis in humans. In: Willoughby, DA and Giroud, JP (eds), *Inflammation: Mechanisms and Treatment.* (Lancaster: MTP Press), pp. 459-66

100. Cutolo, M, Rovida, S, Samanta, E and Accordo, S (1982). Effect of drugs on serum copper and its correlation with other humoral factors in rheumatoid arthritis. In: Willoughby, DA and Giroud, JP (eds), *Inflammation: Mechanisms and Treatment.* (Lancaster: MTP Press), pp. 451-6

101 Rainsford, KD (1982). Environmental metal ion perturbation especially as they affect copper status, are factors in the etiology of arthritic conditions: a hypothesis. In: Sorenson, JRJ (ed), *Inflammatory Diseases and Copper.* (Clifton, NJ: Humana Press), pp. 137-42

102. Klevay, LM (1982). An appraisal of current human copper nutriture. In: Sorenson, JRJ (ed), *Inflammatory Diseases and Copper.* (Clifton, NJ: Humana Press), pp. 123-36

103. Klevay, LM (1981). Relationship between serum, zinc and copper and risk factors associated with cardiovascular disease. *Am J Clin Nutr*, **34**, 597-8

104. Cartwright, GW (1950). In: McElroy, WD and Glass, B (eds), *Copper Metabolism.* (Maryland: Johns Hopkins Press), p274

105. Cartwright, GE and Wintrobe, MM (1964). Copper metabolism in normal subjects. *Am J Clin Nutr*, **14**, 224-32

106. Klevay, LM, Reck, SJ and Barcome, DF (1979). Evidence of dietary copper and zinc deficiencies. *J Am Med Assoc*, **241**, 1916-18

107. Taper, LJ, Hinners, ML and Ritchey, SJ (1982). Effect of zinc intake on copper balance in adult females. *Am J Clin Nutr*, **33**, 1077-82

108. Milne, DB, Schnakenberg, DD, Johnson, HL and Kuhl, GL (1980). Trace mineral intake of enlisted military personnel. Preliminary observations. *J Am Diet Assoc*, **76**, 41-5

109. Ritzmann, SE, Coleman, SL and Levin, WC (1960). The effect of some mercaptanes upon a macrocryogelglobulin; modifications induced by cysteamine, penicillamine and penicillin. *J Clin Invest*, **39**, 1320-9

110. Jaffe, IA (1962). Intra-articular dissociation of the rheumatoid factor. *J Lab Clin Med*, **60**, 409-21

111. Meacock, SCR, Swann, BD and Dawson, W (1981). The dynamics and possible role of metal complexes in inflammation. In: Rainsford, KD, Brune, K and Whitehouse, MW (eds), *Trace Elements in Pathogenesis and Treatment of Inflammation.* (Basel: Birkhauser Verlag), pp.

112. Lipsky, PE and Ziff, M (1978). The effect of D-penicillamine on mitogen-induced human lymphocyte proliferation: synergistic inhibition by D-penicillamine and copper salts. *J Immunol*, **120**, 1006-13

113. Goldberg, LS and Barnett, EV (1970). Essential cryoglobulinemia. Immunologic studies before and after penicillamine therapy. *Arch Intern Med*, **125**, 145-50

114. Bluestone, R and Goldberg, LS (1973). Effect of D-penicillamine on serum immunoglobulins and rheumatoid factor. *Ann Rheum Dis*, **32**, 50-2
115. Jaffe, IA (1963). Comparison of the effects of plasmapheresis and penicillamine on the level of circulating rheumatoid factor. *Ann Rheum Dis*, **22**, 71-6
116. Jaffe, IA (1965). The effect of penicillamine on the laboratory parameters in rheumatoid arthritis. *Arthr Rheum*, **8**, 1064-79
117. Schumacher, K, Maerker-Alzer, G and Preuss, R (1975). Effect of D-penicillamine on lymphocyte function. *Arzneim-Forsch*, **25**, 603-6
118. Tabin, MS and Altman, K (1964). Accelerated immune response induced by D-penicillamine. *Proc Soc Exp Biol Med*, **115**, 225-8
119. Hubner, KF and Gengozian, N (1965). Depression of the primary immune response by D-l-penicillamine. *Proc Soc Exp Biol Med*, **118**, 561-5
120. Schumacher, K, Maerker-Alzer, G and Schaaf, W (1975). Influence of D-penicillamine on the immune response of mice. *Arzneim-Forsch*, **25**, 600-3
121. Liyanage, SP and Currey, HL (1972). Failure of oral D-penicillamine to modify adjuvant arthritis or immune response in the rat. *Ann Rheum Dis*, **31**, 521
122. Jaffe, IA (1970). The treatment of rheumatoid arthritis and necrotizing vasculitis with penicillamine. *Arthr Rheum*, **13**, 436-43
123. Golding, JR, Andrews, FM, Camp, V *et al.* (1973). Controlled trials of penicillamine in severe rheumatoid arthritis. *Ann Rheum Dis*, **32**, 385-6
124. Deshmukh, K and Nimni, ME (1969). A defect in the intramolecular and intermolecular cross-linking of collagen caused by penicillamine. II. Functional groups involved in the interaction process. *J Biol Chem*, **244**, 1787-95
125. Tismann, G, Herbert, V, Go, LT and Brenner, L (1972). Inhibition by penicillamine of DNA and protein synthesis in human bone marrow. *Proc Soc Exp Biol Med*, **139**, 355-63
126. Chwalinska-Sadowska, H and Baum, J (1976). The effect of D-penicillamine on polymorphonuclear leukocyte function. *J Clin Invest*, **58**, 871-9
127. Aposhian, HV (1961). Biochemical and pharmacological properties of the metal-binding agent penicillamine. *Fed Proc*, **20**, 185-8
128. Whitehouse, MW, Field, L, Denke, CW and Ryall, R (1975). Is penicillamine a precursor drug? *Scand J Rheumatol*, **4** (Suppl. 8), 183
129. Walshe, JM (1956). Penicillamine, a new oral therapy for Wilson's disease. *Am J Med*, **21**, 187-93
130. Friedman, M (1977). Chemical basis for pharmacological and therapeutic action of penicillamine. *Proc R Soc Med*, **70** (Suppl. 3), 50-60
131. Lengfelder, E, Fuch, C, Yonner, M and Weser, U (1979). Functional aspects of the superoxide dismutative action of Cu-penicillamine. *Biochem Biophys Acta*, **567**, 492-502
132. Muijsers, AO, Van de Stadt, RJ, Henrichs, AM *et al.* (1984). D-penicillamine in patients with rheumatoid arthritis. Serum levels, pharmacokinetic aspects and correlations with clinical course and side effects. *Arth Rheum*, **27**, 1362-9
133. Merryman, P and Jaffe, IA (1978). Effects of penicillamine on the proliferative response of human lymphocytes. *Proc Soc Exp Biol Med*, **157**, 155-791
134. Amor, B, Avery, C and Degery, A (1980). Tiopronine. New antirheumatic drug in rheumatoid arthritis. *Rev Rheum*, **47**, 157-62
135. Pasero, G, Pellegrini, P, Ciompi, ML *et al.* (1980). Tiopronine; new basic treatment of rheumatoid arthritis. *Rev Rheum*, **47**, 163-8
136. Huskisson, EC, Jaffe, IA, Scott, J and Dieppe, PA (1980). 5-thiopyridoxine in rheumatoid arthritis: Clinical and experimental studies. *Arthr Rheum*, **23**, 106-10
137. Lipsky, PE (1981). Modulation of lymphocyte function by copper thiols. *Agents and Actions*, (Suppl.), **8**, 85-102
138. Zvaifler, NJ (1979). Etiology and pathogenesis of rheumatoid arthritis. In: McCarty, DJ (ed), *Arthritis and Allied Conditions*, 9th ed. (Philadelphia: Lea and Febiger), pp.

139. Krane, SM (1979). Mechanisms of tissue destruction in rheumatoid arthritis. In: McCarty, DJ (ed), *Arthritis and Allied Conditions*, 9th ed. (Philadelphia: Lea and Febiger), pp.

140. Fernandez-Madrid, F (1985). Rheumatoid arthritis. In: Stone, J (ed), *Dermatologic Immunology and Allergy*. (St Louis: CV Mosby), pp. 425-55

141. Lipsky, P and Ziff, M (1982). The mechanism of action of gold and D-penicillamine in rheumatoid arthritis. In: Ziff, M *et al.* (eds), *Advances in Inflammation Research*. (New York: Raven Press, Vol.3, pp. 219-35

142. Perrett, D, Sneddon, W and Stephens, AD (1976). Studies on D-penicillamine metabolism in cystinuria and rheumatoid arthritis: isolation of S-methylpenicillamine. *Biochem Pharmacol*, **25**, 259-64

143. Dormandy, TL (1980). In: *Biological Roles of Copper*. Ciba Foundation Symposium. (Amsterdam: Excerpta Medica), Vol.2, p293

144. Osterberg, R (1980). Therapeutic uses of copper chelating agents. In: *Biological Roles of Copper*. Ciba Foundation Symposium. (Amsterdam: Excerpta Medica), p.283-299

145. Mery, C, Delrieu, F, Ghozlan, R *et al.* (1976). Controlled trial of D-penicillamine in rheumatoid arthritis. *Scand J Rheumatol*, **5**, 241-7

146. Prasad, AS, Brewer, GJ, Schoolmaker, EB and Rabbani, P (1978). Hypocupremia induced by zinc therapy in adults. *J Am Med Assoc*, **240**, 2166-8

147. Fischer, PF, Giroux, A and L'Abbé, MR (1984). Effect of zinc supplementation on copper status in adult man. *Am J Clin Nutr*, **40**, 743-6

6
Copper complexes in the treatment of experimental inflammatory conditions: inflammation, ulcers and pain

JRJ Sorenson
Division of Medicinal Chemistry
University of Arkansas College of Pharmacy
4301 W Markham Street
Little Rock, Arkansas 72205, USA

I. INTRODUCTION

Copper, like sodium, potassium, magnesium, calcium, iron, zinc, chromium, vanadium, and manganese, is an essential metalloelement and as such it is required by all human cells for normal metabolism[1]. However, some cells have greater metabolic needs than others and tissue content reflects this fact. Amounts of copper found in various body tissues and fluids of individuals, who died sudden accidental deaths[2,3], are shown in Table 1.

The amount of copper in each tissue correlates with the number and kind of metabolic processes requiring copper. In this regard, it is of interest to point out that brain and heart contain more copper than all other tissues except the liver, which is a major copper storage organ. Gall bladder and bile also contain large amounts of copper which has been attributed to their supposed roles in excretion. However, the gall bladder may also serve as a storage tissue and bile may contain a mobile storage form of copper suitable for intestinal reabsorption. The large kidney copper content, when compared with the very small urine copper content, suggests a conservatory role for the kidney. Gastric and intestinal tissues also have high copper contents, and this reflects their high metabolic rates. Remaining tissues have lesser amounts of copper because of their relatively lower metabolic activity but it is just as important for normal metabolism in these tissues as it is in all others.

Although bile may serve as the major excretory vehicle for excess copper, significant but lesser amounts are lost via hair, stratum corneum, finger- and toe-nails, sweat, and urine as end-products of metabolism. These losses

Copper and Zinc in Inflammation. Milanino, R, Rainsford, KD and Velo, GP (eds)
Inflammation and Drug Therapy Series, Volume IV

point out the need for compensating daily intake of 3 mg *and absorption* to replenish daily losses of this essential metalloelement.

Table 1 Mean concentrations⃰ of Cu in tissue and fluids[2,3]

Adrenal	210	Muscle	85
Aorta	97	Nails	23 μg/g
Bile	547	Oesophagus	140
Blood (total)	1.01 μg/ml	Omentum	190
erythrocytes	0.98 μg/ml	Ovary	130
plasma	1.12 μg/ml	Pancreas	150
serum	1.19 μg/ml	Pancreatic fluid	105
Bone	25 μg/g	Placenta	4 μg/g
Brain	370	Prostate	110
Breast	6 μg/g	Saliva	0.08 μg/ml
Cerebrospinal fluid	0.22 μg/g	Skin	120
Diaphragm	150	Spleen	93
Gallbladder	750	Stomach	230
Hair	19 μg/g	Sweat	0.55 μg/ml
Heart	350	Testes	95
Intestine		Thymus	4 μg/g
duodenum	300	Thyroid	100
jejunum	250	Tongue	4.6 μg/g
ileum	280	Tooth	
cecum	220	dentine	2 μg/g
sigmoid colon	230	enamel	10 μg/g
rectum	180	Trachea	65
Kidney	270	Urinary bladder	120
Larynx	59	Urine	0.04 μg/ml
Liver	680	Uterus	110
Lung	130		
Lymph node	60		
Milk			
colostrum	0.35-0.50 μg/ml		
mature	0.20-0.50 μg/ml		

⃰ μg/g of tissue ash or as shown

Ionic copper has a particularly high affinity for other molecules (ligands) capable of bonding with it. A consequence of this is that all measurable copper in biological systems exists as complexes or chelates composed of copper bonded to organic components of these systems. Calculated amounts of ionic copper suggested to be present in biological systems (10^{-18} M in plasma[4]) are too small to be measured using the most sensitive instrumentation available. As a result, measurable tissue copper content reflects content of copper complexes, and these complexes account for the absorption, distribution, and biologically active forms, including copper-dependent enzymes.

Table 2 Recognized copper-dependent enzymes and their chemical function

Enzyme	Function
Cytochrome c oxidase	Reduction of oxygen: $O_2 \to HO_2 \to H_2O_2 \to H_2O + HO \to H_2O$
Superoxide dismutase	Disproportionation of superoxide in prevention of its accumulation: $2O_2^- + 2H^+ \to O_2 + H_2O_2$
Tyrosinase	Hydroxylation of tyrosine in melanin synthesis:
Dopamine-β-hydroxylase and extremely acidic copper-containing protein	Hydroxylation of dopamine in catecholamine synthesis:
Lysyl oxidase	Oxidation of terminal amino group of lysyl amino acids in procollagen and proelastin to an aldehyde group: $R\text{-}CH_2\text{-}CH_2\text{-}NH_2 \to R\text{-}CH_2\text{-}CH = O$
Amine oxidases	Oxidation of primary amines to aldehydes in catecholamine and other primary amine metabolism: $R\text{-}CH_2\text{-}NH_2 \to R\text{-}CH = O$
Caeruloplasmin	Mobilization and utilization of stored iron: Ferroxidase Fe(II) $\to$ Fe(III) "Angiogenin"
Factor V	Blood clotting
Peptidyl α-amidating	Synthesis of neuroendocrine peptides (hypothalmic thyrotropin releasing hormone, α-melanocyte stimulating hormone from anterior pituitary, gastrin from stomach, and choleocystokinin from the small intestine): Peptidyl-NH-CH$_2$COOH $\to$ peptidyl-NH$_2$ + O = CHCOOH

For the tyrosine hydroxylation reaction, the structures show tyrosine being converted to dihydroxyphenylalanine.

For the dopamine hydroxylation reaction, dopamine is converted to Norepinephrine.

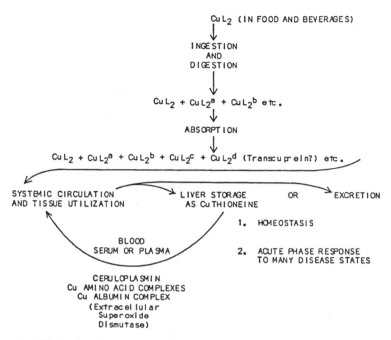

Figure 1 Distribution of copper complexes following ingestion, digestion, and absorption.

Recognised and recently suggested copper-dependent enzymes[5-14] are listed in Table 2, along with their functions. In addition, copper-dependent processes appear to be required for modulation of prostaglandin syntheses, lysosomal membrane stabilization, and modulation of histaminic activity[15]. Ingested copper complexes representing the recommended 3 mg (47 μmol) daily intake of copper follow the pathway presented in Figure 1. One of a large number of possible copper complexes that might be found in foods and/or beverages (CuL_2), following ingestion and digestion, would give rise to the formation of other copper complexes as a result of exchange with ligands (L) in the enzyme digest (amino acids, fatty acids, amines, etc.) or ternary complexes of the original complex. Ternary complexes are complexes formed by the addition of another ligand, such as a small peptide or amino acid, to an existing complex to form a new complex having a larger molecular mass. It is important to remember that gastric digestion is enzyme catalysed and not acid catalysed and, since gastric pH is likely to range from 6 to 3 with the ingestion of a meal[16], as shown in Figure 2, some of the originally ingested complex may be absorbed intact. Copper complexes in the duodenal chyme (pH 7.0), Figure 2, would also be expected to be absorbed intact. It is also worth noting that pharmacological doses of copper complexes have an antisecretory effect and thus prevent lowering of the normal empty stomach pH (6.0).

Additional complexes such as transcuprein[17] (Figure 1), which may be a ternary complex of an absorbed smaller complex, or a ternary albumin complex may also be formed, without ligand exchange, following systemic absorption. Again, depending upon the concentration absorbed, some of the original complex may remain intact in plasma. All of these copper complexes then undergo systemic circulation to all tissues and are: (1) utilized by tissues following ligand exchange with apoenzymes and apoproteins to form metalloenzymes and metalloproteins, (2) stored in the liver following ligand exchange with thioneine to form copper-thioneine, or (3) excreted in the event tissue needs have been met and stores replenished. Since excessive copper storage has never been reported in any normal population, and copper complex absorption must vary in these populations, efficient homeostatic mechanisms must regulate retention and excretion of varying amounts of absorbed copper complexes in all normal, non-Wilson's disease, individuals.

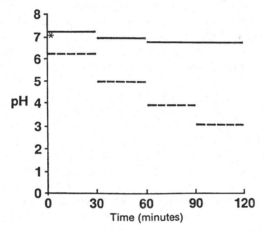

Figure 2 Change in pH of chyme entering the duodenum (- - -) and leaving the duodenum (——) following the ingestion of a pH 7.1 meal (*) (adapted from Davenport[16]).

Also shown in Figure 1, copper-thioneine-stored copper is released from the liver as complexed forms; ceruloplasmin, copper amino acid complexes, and a copper albumin complex, to meet normal metabolic needs. This homeostatic release of copper complexes from the liver meets normal copper-dependent physiological requirements of body tissues including *de novo* synthesis of copper-dependent enzymes.

The essentiality of copper is now understood based upon its recognized need for activation of copper-dependent enzymes. Complexed forms of copper also facilitate absorption, tissue distribution, and tissue utilization. In the non-disease state these forms of copper account for the physiological regulation of copper-dependent homeostatic processes. Since copper is needed for normal metabolism and prevention of disease, great care should be taken to assure that dietary intake provides required amounts of copper. Unfortunately, many or nearly all modern diets studied[18] do not supply required amounts of this and other essential metalloelements. It is then reasonable to suggest that marginal or deficient intakes or impaired absorption may lead to decreased enzyme activity and manifestations of acute inflammatory disease in the short term as well as manifestations of chronic inflammatory disease in the long term.

II. ANTI-INFLAMMATORY ACTIVITIES OF COPPER COMPLEXES

Larger than normal concentrations of blood copper complexes are associated with various chronic inflammatory disease states[15], and it is likely that this association exists for acute and chronic gastrointestinal ulcer diseases which are, in part, inflammatory diseases of gastric or intestinal tissues. The elevation usually found in inflammatory diseases is generally two to three times the normal concentration during the active disease phase. With disease remission plasma copper complex concentrations return to normal.

The central question concerning this observation is whether the elevation is a cause of the disease or a response to the disease. Many interpret elevated concentrations of blood copper complexes as a cause of inflammatory disease. It is equally plausible that this elevation is a physiological response to inflammatory disease. Since there is no evidence that elevation of normal blood copper-containing components causes any of these diseases, the hypothesis that elevation of plasma copper-containing components is a general physiological response to inflammatory diseases merits serious consideration. The fact that small molecular weight copper complexes have anti-inflammatory activity in man[19] and animal models of inflammation is offered as evidence that the associated increase in blood copper-containing components is a physiological response which has a role in mediating remission when remission occurs.

To date, over 70 copper complexes have been studied as anti-inflammatory agents. Results of these studies, which have been reviewed[15], confirm as well as extend original observations that copper complexes are the active metabolites of anti-arthritic drugs[20].

As shown in Table 3, $Cu(II)_2(acetate)_4$ was found to be active in the initial test (carrageenan paw oedema) for anti-inflammatory screens (cotton wad granuloma and adjuvant arthritis). Copper chloride had no activity in any of these models of inflammation at the initial screening doses of 1.18, 0.59, and 0.18 mmol/kg respectively. Ligands such as anthranilic acid and 3,5-diisopropylsalicylic acid (3,5-dips) which were anticipated to be inactive were found to be inactive. However, their copper complexes were found to be potent anti-inflammatory agents in all three models of inflammation. These observations support the notion that complexed copper is a more active anti-inflammatory form of copper, and led to the suggestion that copper complexes of active anti-inflammatory agents might be more active than their parent anti-inflammatory drugs.

Table 3 Anti-inflammatory activities of some copper complexes

Compound	Carrageenan paw oedema	Cotton wad granuloma	Adjuvant arthritis	Copper (%)
$Cu(II)_2(acetate)_4H_2O)_2$	A[b] at 0.02	I[c] at 0.30	I at 0.089	31.8
anthranilic acid	I at 1.46	NT[d]	I at 0.219	
3,5-dips acid	I at 0.90	NT	I at 0.135	
$Cu(II)(anthranilate)_2$	A at 0.02	A at 0.07	A at 0.003	18.9
$Cu(II)(3,5,dips)_2$	A at 0.02	A at 0.01	A at 0.002	12.5
Aspirin	A at 0.36	A at 1.11(i.g.)	A at 0.033	
$Cu(II)_2(aspirinate)_4$	A at 0.01	A at 0.01	A at 0.001	15.0
D-penicillamine	I at 1.34	I at 0.67	I at 0.201	
$Cu(I)(D-pen)(H_2O)1.5$	A at 0.03	A at 0.04	NT	26.7
$Cu(II)_2(D-pen disulfide)_2(H_2O)_2$	A at 0.01	A at 0.03	A at 0.040[e]	15.4

[a]All compounds were given by subcutaneous injection unless indicated as intragastric (i.g.) and expressed as millimole per kilogram of body weight (mmol/kg); [b]lowest active dose tested; [c]inactive; [d]not tested; [e]only dose of this penicillamine complex tested.

Representative data from the original report comparing aspirin, a standard in arthritis therapy, and D-penicillamine, an arthritic disease-modifying agent, with their copper complexes are also presented in Table 3. These data show that $Cu(II)_2(aspirinate)_4$ is at least 30 times as effective as aspirin, and copper complexes of penicillamine are many times more effective than penicillamine. These results, along with data provided by many others[15], support the hypothesis that active metabolites of anti-arthritic drugs are their copper complexes. Since amounts of copper in these complexes (Table 3) do not appear to correlate with activity, it is suggested that pharmacological activity may be better correlated with the physicochemical properties of these copper complexes.

Acute toxicity studies were done early in the course of this work[20,21]. These studies demonstrated that anti-inflammatory copper complexes were less toxic than inorganic forms of copper, as well as their parent anti-arthritic drugs. The oral LD_{50} values for Cu $(II)_2(aspirinate)_4$ were found to be 1.06 ± 0.26 and 1.16 ± 0.33 mmol/kg, respectively, for male and female Sprague-Dawley rats. Chronic toxicity studies using 0.12 mmol (100 mg)/kg given orally to Sprague-Dawley rats 5 days per week for 3 months did not affect growth, survival, plasma copper or zinc concentrations, or copper and zinc concentrations in 15 tissues including skin and fur[22]. Histopathological examination of all tissues, except skin and fur, at the light microscopic level revealed no evidence of pathological changes except for an increase in Kupffer cell number in the liver of those animals that were sacrificed at the end of the 3-month treatment period. Kupffer cell number progressively decreased in liver of animals sacrificed at the end of the subsequent 2 months of this 5-month study. The projected human dose of $Cu(II)_2(aspirinate)_4$ is 3 to 6 µmol/kg daily with a decrease to some maintenance dose with remission. This regimen seems to be safe enough since the recommended safe intake of copper is 47 µmol/day.

Two general chemical mechanisms are immediately apparent possibilities. Small molecular weight copper complexes may serve as transport forms of copper that allow activation of copper-dependent enzymes, or they may have chemical reactivities that facilitate correction of the chemical problem that led to the disease state. Activation of peptidyl lysyl oxidase which is ultimately required to catalyze cross-linking of connective tissue components in the tissue repair phase of anti-inflammatory action is an important mechanistic consideration in accounting for anti-inflammatory activity of copper complexes[15]. Activation of the copper-dependent superoxide dismutases (Cu-ZnSOD) which are required to prevent accumulation of superoxide and subsequent synthesis of oxyradicals, as a result of reduced Cu-ZnSOD activity, has been suggested as the cause of arthritic and other inflammatory diseases[13-15]. Since small molecular weight copper complexes have been shown to disproportionate superoxide[14,15] this chemical reactivity of copper complexes has attracted a great deal of attention in accounting for anti-inflammatory activity of copper complexes[15]. Other less well understood possible mechanisms involve modulation of inflammation mediators such as histamine, lysosomal membrane stabilization, and prostaglandin syntheses[15].

Anti-inflammatory activities of copper complexes partially explain the earlier observations by Fenz, Forestier, Kuzell, and Hangarter that copper complexes are effective in treating arthritic and other human degenerative diseases[19]. Another partial explanation comes from the observation that copper complexes have potent analgesic activity.

III. ANALGESIC ACTIVITIES OF COPPER COMPLEXES

It has very recently been reported that copper complexes of non-steroidal anti-inflammatory agents are more effective analgesics that their parent drugs[23]. As shown in Table 4, copper complexes of salicylic acid, 3,5-dips, aspirin, niflumic acid, and indomethacin were more effective analgesics than their parent compounds and copper chloride or copper acetate. In addition, the copper complex of indomethacin was found to be as effective as morphine in both pain models and the amount of copper in the 1 µmol dose of $Cu(II)_2(indomethacin)_4$ is one-fiftieth the recommended safe daily intake of copper. These data support the hypothesis that copper complexes are the active forms, formed *in vivo*, of the non-steroidal anti-inflammatory agents and the hypothesis that these complexes activate opioid receptors[23].

Table 4 Analgesic effects of parent ligands and copper complexes on acetic acid-induced writhing pain in mice and adjuvant-induced arthritis pain in rats

Compound	Doses[a] (mmol/kg)	% inhib.	ED_{50}(mmol/kg) (95% C.L.)	Doses[a] (mmol/kg)	% inhib.	ED_{50} (mmol/kg) (95% C.L.)
		Writhing pain			*Arthritic pain*	
Salicylic acid	2.17	38*	>2.17	0.72	33	1.83
				1.44	43	(0.49-6.81)
				2.88	60	
Cu(II)$_2$(salicylate)$_4$	0.30	20	1.53	0.15	30	0.25
	0.59	27	(0.61-3.80)	0.30	47	(0.13-0.48)
	1.18	46*		0.59	90	
3,5-Dips	0.22	19	0.4	0.45	27	>0.90
	0.45	56**	(0.29-0.67)	0.90	43	
	0.90	78***				
Cu(II)(3,4-dips)$_2$	0.20	26	0.43	0.40	40	>0.40
	0.40	56*	(0.20-0.91)			
	0.79	62***				
Aspirin	0.21	32	0.48	0.56	30	1.41
	0.42	41*	(0.22-1.04)	1.11	40	(0.50-3.96)
	0.84	67***		2.22	63	
Cu(II)$_2$(aspirinate)$_4$	0.09	32*	0.14	0.03	13	0.09
	0.18	59**	(0.09-0.25)	0.06	30	(0.04-0.21)
	0.36	80***		0.12	60	
Niflumic acid	0.13	38*	0.21	0.18	23	0.48
	0.27	51**	(0.11-0.40)	0.35	43	(0.19-1.20)
	0.53	80***		0.71	60	
Cu(II)$_2$(niflumate)$_4$	0.06	33*	0.10	0.16	37	>0.16
	0.12	57***	(0.05-0.20)			
	0.24	73***				
Indomethacin	0.007	27	0.01	0.007	23	0.02
	0.014	60**	(0.01-0.03)	0.014	43	(0.01-0.03)
	0.028	68***		0.028	70	
Cu(II)$_2$(indomethacin)$_4$	0.001	38	0.002	0.001	20	0.002
	0.002	53**	(0.001-0.003)	0.002	40	(0.001-0.003)
	0.004	75***		0.003	87	
Cu(II)(chloride)$_2$				2.24	0	>2.24
Cu(II)$_2$(acetate)$_4$				0.83	0	>0.83
Morphine HCl[b]	0.001	35	0.002	0.001	20	0.002
	0.002	44*	(0.001-0.003)	0.002	40	(0.001-0.005)
	0.004	89***		0.004	60	

[a]administered orally in 5% propylene glycol and 1.4% polyvinyl alcohol in water; [b]administered subcutaneously in saline; *p < 0.05; **p < 0.01; ***p < 0.001 versus vehicle-treated group.

IV. ANTI-ULCER ACTIVITIES OF COPPER COMPLEXES

Based upon observations that copper complexes appeared to facilitate the synthesis of superior granuloma around cotton pellets in the cotton wad granuloma model of inflammation, it was hypothesized that these complexes promoted connective tissue synthesis, as in wound repair, in response to inflammatory insults. To examine this possibility these copper complexes were evaluated as anti-ulcer agents.

Copper complexes were subsequently found to be potent anti-ulcer agents in the Shay and corticoid-induced models of ulcer[20]. To date, over 60 copper compounds have been shown to have anti-ulcer activity in six different models of gastric ulcer[15]. Representative data from the original report[20] are presented in Table 5.

Table 5 Oral anti-ulcer activity of non-steroidal anti-inflammatory agent copper complexes

Compound	Anti-ulcer activity (μmol//kg)	Percentage copper
$Cu(II)_2(acetate)_4(H_2O)_2$	53	32
$Cu(II)(anthranilate)_2$	13	19
$Cu(II)_2(aspirinate)_4$	13	15
$Cu(II)(salicylate)_2.8H_2O$	11	15
$Cu(II)(fenamole)_2(HCl)_2$	10	14
$Cu(II)_2(fenamole)_2(acetate)_4$	7	19
$Cu(II)(butazolidine)_2$	7	9
$Cu(II)_2(D-pen\ disulfide)_2.3H_2O$	6	16
$Cu(II)(3,5-dips)_2$	5	13
$Cu(II)_2(niflumate)_4$	4	10
$Cu(II)_2(indomethacin)_4$	3	8

Copper(II)$_2$(acetate)$_4$ had only very weak anti-ulcer activity. However, copper complexes of the non-steroidal anti-inflammatory agents were found to be potent anti-ulcer agents. There are no more potent anti-ulcer agents in this model of ulcer. From data presented in Table 5 it is also clear that anti-ulcer activity is not directly related to copper content. It is most likely that anti-ulcer activity is related to the physiochemical properties of these complexes. It is also worth noting that the amount of copper in these ED$_{50}$ doses represents one-fourth to one-fifteenth of the recommended daily intake of copper.

A subsequent comparison of the relative anti-ulcer activities of three different penicillamine complexes in the Shay ulcer model revealed that the water-soluble mixed valence complex, $Na_5Cu(I)_8Cu(II)_6$ (penicillamine)$_{12}Cl$, was the most effective[24]. Copper complexes of amino acids have also been found to be effective in preventing Shay ulcers and reducing the severity of the remaining gastric lesions[25,26]. The copper complex of glycine was the most effective of all of the amino acid complexes studied, and it was essentially as effective as propantheline in reducing ulcer number as well as ulcer severity[25].

In our original report of anti-ulcer activity for copper complexes we also reported that these copper complexes reduced gastric acid secretion in the Shay rat[20]. The influence of copper complexes on histamine activity was examined by studying the activity of the copper complex of histamine. Copper(II)(histamine)(Cl$_2$) was found to be a potent *anti-ulcer* and *anti-secretory* agent. This observation was confirmed and extended by Marletta *et al.*[27] and Alberghina *et al.*[28] with reports that the mixed copper complex of tryptophan and phenylalanine, Cu(II)(Try)(Phe), inhibited histamine-, pentagastrin-, and bethanacol-induced gastric acid secretion in the Shay rat. Its ED$_{50}$ in reducing gastric acid secretion in the non-stimulated Shay rat was 77 ± 7 μmol/kg when it was administered intragastrically 1 h before ligation[28].

Table 6 Comparison of Cu(II)(salicylate)$_2$ and cimetidine, given orally, in protecting against gastric lesions produced by oral ulcerogenic doses of aspirin (2.22 mmol/kg), indomethacin (56 μmol/kg), and cold-stress in rats

Ulcerogen	Anti-ulcer agent	Dose (μmol/kg)	% inhibition (M $\pm$ SE)
Aspirin	Cimetidine	148	19 ± 5
		297	16 ± 4
	Cu(II)(salicylate)$_2$	22	21 ± 6
		44	61 ± 10^a
Indomethacin	Cimetidine	148	10 ± 3
		297	24 ± 6
	Cu(II)(salicylate)$_2$	22	37 ± 7^a
		44	50 ± 5^a
Cold-Stress	Cimetidine	148	38 ± 8^a
		297	61 ± 9^a
	Cu(II)(salicylate)$_2$	22	58 ± 8^a
		44	79 ± 7^a

[a]Significant at p < 0.05 (when compared with values obtained for non-treated rats)

These observations were confirmed and extended by West and his colleages with reports showing that Cu(II)$_2$(aspirinate)$_4$ and Cu(II)(salicylate)$_2$ were more effective in the aspirin-exacerbated Shay ulcer model than either the H$_1$(mepyramine) or H$_2$(metiamide) histamine blockers[28]. It was also shown that Cu(II)(salicylate)$_2$ was more effective than these anti-histaminic compounds and cimetidine in the cold-stress ulcer model[29,30] and Cu(II)(salicylate)$_2$ was more effective than cimetidine in preventing aspirin and indomethacin-induced ulcers (Table 6)[30]. Finally, Townsend demonstrated that Cu(II)(tryptophan)$_2$ and Cu(II)$_2$(aspirinate)$_4$ increased the rate of healing of surgically placed glandular gastric ulcers using histochemical methods[31]. These complexes prevented wound regression, increased the rate of re-epithelialization, and replaced connective tissue components could not be distinguished from tissue of normal non-operated rats. Townsend also found that treatment with these copper complexes prevented spleen, pancreas, and liver adhesions to the stomach, a constant feature associated with non-treated surgically placed glandular gastric ulcers.

The originally reported anti-secretory activity of copper complexes[20] has, at least in part, been explained as anti-histaminic activity or as a modulation of histamine activity[25-30]. This suggestion is consistent with observations that copper markedly increases (50-fold) specific cimetidine bonding to brain membrane H$_2$ receptors[32-34] and that copper decreases compound 48/80 and concanavalin-A induced releases of histamine from peritoneal mast cells[35]. Further explanation of the anti-secretory effect comes from the work of Boyle et al. [36] showing that the anti-ulcer anti-secretory activity of non-steroidal anti-inflammatory agent copper complexes modulate syntheses of prostaglandins E$_2$ and F$_{2\alpha}$, which is consistent with other reports of copper complex modulation of prostaglandin syntheses[37-41].

Superoxide dismutase-mimetic activity of anti-ulcer copper complexes[42-50] also offers an accounting of the reduction in number of ulcers[20,24,26,29,30], reduced severity of remaining ulcers[24-25], and the apparent absence of wound regression in treated surgically placed gastric wounds[31]. Superoxide dismutase mimetic activity of Cu(II)(3,5-dips)$_2$ was also used to account for its abolition of desoxycholate-induced colonic epithelial proliferation, and to suggest an oxyradical aetiology for inflammatory bowel disease[51]. Based upon these observations it seems reasonable to suggest that a reduction in intestinal and gastric tissue copper-dependent superoxide dismutase (Cu-ZnSOD) and the accumulation of superoxide and other oxyradicals have an aetiologic or pathogenic role in gastric and intestinal ulceration. Lipophilic copper complexes may be effective in crossing lipid cell membranes and either inducing or facilitating *de novo* synthesis of Cu-ZnSOD or dismutating superoxide as a result of their own chemical reactivity.

Maintenance and repair of duodenal and gastric collagen and elastin connective tissue components also seems to be an important copper-dependent enzyme function in preventing or repairing duodenal or gastric ulcers. Induction or facilitation *de novo* synthesis of peptidyl lysyl oxidase by copper complexes[52] merits consideration in accounting for the observed rapid and normal replacement of connective tissue components in the surgically placed gastric ulcer model[31].

Recently recognised roles for copper-dependent peptidyl α-amidating enzymes in intestinal and gastric tissues for syntheses of choleocystokinin and gastrin, respectively, may also be important in understanding normal gastrointestinal physiology as well as accounting for anti-ulcer activity of copper complexes[11].

Potent anti-ulcer activity without ulcerogenic activity[33] coupled with potent anti-inflammatory and analgesic activities distinguishes copper complexes as a unique class of anti-inflammatory agents since all other anti-inflammatory drugs do not have anti-ulcer activity but are ulcerogenic. A search for more bio-effective copper complexes would seem to be a much more valid approach to developing more effective anti-arthritic drugs rather than searching for selective copper chelating agents[54,55] which has in the past led to the development of the currently used less effective and more toxic anti-arthritic drugs. All of the above mechanistic considerations offer support for the possibility that pharmacological uses of copper complexes represent a physiological approach to treatment of inflammation, ulcers, and pain.

Acknowledgements

I am indebted to the International Copper Research Association, Max and Victoria Dreyfus Foundation, Denver Roller Corporation, and the Elsa U. Pardee Foundation for financial support enabling the writing of this manuscript.

References

1. Underwood, EJ (1977).*Trace Elements in Human and Animal Nutrition*, 3rd edn. (New York: Academic Press)
2. Tipton, IH and Cook, MJ (1963). Trace elements in human tissue. II: Adult subjects from the United States.*Health Phys*, 1, 103-145
3. Iyengar, GV, Kollmer, WE and Bowen, HJM (1978).*The Elemental Composition of Tissue and Body Fluids*. (New York: Springer)
4. May, PM, Linder, PW and Williams, DR (1976). Ambivalent effect of protein binding on computed distribution of metal ions complexed by ligands in blood plasma.*Experientia*, **32**, 1492-1493
5. Boyadzhyan, AS (1985). Purification of dopamine-β-monoxygenase and the extremely acidic copper-containing protein from the adrenal medulla: the extremely acidic copper-containing protein as an electron donor for dopamine-β-monooxygenase. *Biochemistry*, **50**, 75-81
6. Frieden, E (1986). Perspectives on copper biochemistry. *Clin Physiol Biochem*, **4**, 11-19
7. O'Dell, BL (1976). Biochemistry and physiology of copper in vertebrates. In Prasad, AS and Oberleas, D (eds), *Trace Elements in Human Health and Disease, Vol.I, Zinc and Copper*, 391-413 (New York: Academic Press)
8. McCord, JM and Fridovich, I (1969). Superoxide dismutase. An enzymatic function for erythrocuprein (hemocuprein). *J Biol Chem*, **244**, 6049-6055
9. Fridovich, I (1986). Biological effects of the superoxide radical. *Arch Biochem Biophys*, **247**, 1-11

10. Hamilton, GA (1981). Oxidases with monocopper reactive sites. In Spiro, TG (ed), *Copper Proteins*, 193-218 (New York: Wiley)

11. Anonymous (1985). Newly found roles for copper. *Nutr Rev*, **43**, 117-119

12. Marklund, S, Holme, E and Hellner, L (1982). Superoxide dismutase in extracellular fluids. *Clin Chem Acta*, **126**, 41-51

13. Marklund, S (1984). Extracellular-superoxide dismutase in human tissues and human cell-lines. *J Clin Acta*, **74**, 1398-1403

14. Sorenson, JRJ, Oberley, LW, Crouch, RK and Kensler, TW (1984). Pharmacologic activities of SOD-like copper complexes. In Bors, W, Saran, M and Tait, D (eds), *Oxygen Radicals in Chemistry and Biology*, 821-830 (Berlin: Walter de Gruyter and Co)

15. Sorenson, JRJ (1976). The antiinflammatory activities of copper complexes. In Siegel, H (ed), *Metal Ions in Biological Systems*, 77-124 (New York: Marcel Dekker)

16. Davenport, HC (1982). *Physiology of the Digestive Tract*, 5th edn, 132-133 (Chicago: Year Book Medical Publishers)

17. Weiss, KC and Linder, MC (1985). Copper transport in rats involving a new plasma protein. *Am J Physiol*, **249**, E77-E88

18. Sorenson, JRJ, Oberley, LW, Kishore, V, *et al.* (1984). Copper complexes: a physiologic approach to the treatment of 'inflammatory diseases'. *Inorg Chim Acta*, **91**, 285-294

19. Sorenson, JRJ and Hangarter, W (1977). Treatment of rheumatoid and degenerative diseases with copper complexes. *Inflammation*, **2**, 217-238

20. Sorenson, JRJ (1976). Copper complexes as possible active forms of the antiarthritic agents. *J Med Chem*, **19**, 135-148

21. Sorenson, JRJ (1978). Copper complexes, a unique class of antiarthritic drugs. *Prog Med Chem*, **15**, 211-260

22. Sorenson, JRJ, Rolniak, TM and Chang, LW (1984). Preliminary chronic toxicity study of copper aspirinate. *Inorg Chim Acta*, **91**, L31-34

23. Okuyama, S, Hashimoto, S, Aihara, H, *et al.* (1987). Copper complexes of non-steroidal antiinflammatory agents: analgestic activity and possible opioid receptor activation. *Agents and Actions*, **21**, 130-144

24. Sorenson, JRJ, Ramakrishna, K and Rolniak, TM (1982). Actiulcer activity of D-penicillamine copper complexes. *Agents and Actions*, **12**, 408-411

25. Kishore, V, Rolniak, TM, Ramakrishna, K and Sorenson, JRJ (1982). The antiulcer activities of copper complexes. In Sorenson, JRJ (ed), *Inflammatory Diseases and Copper*, 363-373 (Clifton, NJ: Humana Press)

26. West, GB (1982). The copper problem and amino acids. In Sorenson, JRJ (ed), *Inflammatory Diseases and Copper*, 319-327 (Clifton, NJ: Humana Press)

27. Marletta, F, Rizzarelli, E, Mangiameli, A, *et al.* (1977). Atti XXI Congress Naz Soc Ital Gastroenterol, Bologna, 1977; *Rendic Gastroenterol*, **9** (Suppl 1) 35

28. Alberghina, M, Brogna, A, Mangiamelli, J, *et al.* (1982). Copper (II) complexes of amino acids: gastric acid anti-secretory activity in rats. *Il Farmaco*, **12**, 805-814

29. Hayden, LJ, Thomas, C and West, GB (1978). Inhibitors of gastric lesions in the rat. *J Pharm Pharmacol*, **30**, 244-246

30. West, GB (1982). Testing for drugs inhibiting the formation of gastric ulcers. *J Pharmacol Methods*, **8**, 33-37

31. Townsend, SF and Sorenson, JRJ (1981). Effect of copper aspirinate on regeneration of gastric mucosa following surgical lesions. In Rainsford, KD, Brune, K and Whitehouse, MW (eds), *Trace Elements in the Pathogenesis and Treatment of Inflammatory Conditions*, 389-398 (Basel: Birkhauser Verlag)

32. Kendall, DA, Ferkany, JW and Enna, SJ (1980). Properties of ^{3}H-cimetidine binding in rat brain membranes. *Fed Proc*, **39**, 390

33. Kendall, DA, Ferkany, JW and Enna, SJ (1980). Properties of ^{3}H-cimetidine binding in rat brain membrane fractions. *Life Sci*, **26**, 1293-1302

34. Kawai, M, Nomura, Y and Segawa, T (1984). Elevation of [^{3}H]cimetidine binding by CuCl$_2$ in brain membranes of rats. *Neurochem Int*, **6**, 563-568

35. Jande, MB and Sharma, SC (1986). The effect of cupric sulfate on compound 48/80 and concanavalin-A induced release of histamine from rat peritoneal mast cells. *Br J Pharmacol*, **89**, 570P

36. Boyle, E, Freeman, PC, Goudie, AC *et al.* (1976). Role of copper in preventing gastrointestinal damage by acidic anti-inflammatory drugs. *J Pharm Pharmacol*, **28**, 865-868

37. Lee, RE and Lands, WEM (1972). Cofactors in biosynthesis of prostaglandins F1-alpha and F2-alpha. *Biochim Biophys Acta*, **260**, 203-211

38. Maddox, IS (1973). Role of copper in prostaglandin synthesis. *Biochim Biophys Acta*, **306**, 74-81

39. Vargaftig, BB, Tranier, Y and Chignard, M (1975). Blockade by metal complexing agents and by catalase of effects of arachidonic acid on platelets-relevance to study of antiinflammatory mechanisms. *Eur J Pharmacol*, **33**, 19-29

40. Swift, A, Karmazyn, M, Horrobin, DF *et al.* (1978). Low prostaglandin concentrations cause cardiac rhythm disturbances: effect reversed by low levels of copper or chloroquine. *Prostaglandins*, **15**, 651-657

41. Cunnane, SC, Zinner, H, Horrobin, DF *et al.* (1979). Copper inhibits pressor responses to noradrenaline but not potassium: interactions with prostaglandins E$_1$, E$_2$ and I$_2$ and penicillamine. *Can J Physiol Pharmacol*, **57**, 35-40

42. Brigelius, R, Spottl, R, Bors, W *et al.* (1974). Superoxide dismutase activity of low molecular weight Cu$_2$ plus-chelates studied by pulse radiolysis. *FEBS Lett*, **47**, 72-75

43. Brigelius, R, Hartman, HJ, Bors, W *et al.* (1975). Superoxide dismutase activity of Cu(Tyr)2, and Cu,Co-Erythrocuprein. *Hoppe-Seylers Z Physiol Chem*, **356**, 739-745

44. Paschen, E and Weser, U (1975). Problems concerning the biological action of superoxide dismutase (erythrocuprein). *Hoppe Seylers Z Physiol Chem*, **356**, 727-737

45. DeAlvare, LR, Goda, K and Kimura, T (1976). Mechanisms of superoxide anion scavenging reaction by bis(salicylato)copper(II) complex. *Biochem Biophys Res Commun*, **69**, 687-694

46. Weser, U, Richter, C, Wendel, A and Younes, M (1978). Reactivity of antiinflammatory and superoxide dismutase active Cu(II)-salicylates. *Bioinorg Chem*, **8**, 201-213

47. Younes, M and Weser, U (1977). Superoxide dismutase activity of copper-penicillamine: possible involvement of Cu(I) stabilized sulfur radical. *Biochem Biophys Res Commun*, **78**, 1247-1253

48. Lengfelder, E and Elstner, EF (1978). Determination of the superoxide dismutasing activity of D-penicillamine copper. *Hoppe-Seyler's Z Physiol Chem*, **359**, 751-757

49. Lengfelder, E, Fuchs, C, Younes, M and Weser, U (1979). Functional aspects of the superoxide dismutative action of Cu-penicillamine. *Biochim Biophys Acta*, **567**, 492-502

50. Richardson, T (1976). Salicylates, copper complexes, free radicals, and arthritis. *J Pharm Pharmacol*, **28**, 666

51. Craven, PA, Pfanstiel, J and DeRubertis, FR (1986). Role of reactive oxygen in bile salt stimulation of colonic epithelial proliferation. *J Clin Invest*, **77**, 850-859

52. Harris, ED, DeSilvestro, RA and Balthrop, JE (1982). Lysyl oxidase, a molecular target of copper. In Sorenson, JRJ (ed), *Inflammatory Diseases and Copper*, 183-198 (Clifton, NJ: Humana Press)

53. Williams, DA, Walz, DT and Foye, WO (1976). Synthesis and biological evaluation of tetrakis-μ-Acetylsalicylatodicopper(II). *J Pharm Sci*, **65**, 126-128

54. Milanino, R, Cassini, A, Franco, L *et al.* (1985). Copper metabolism in the acute inflammatory process and its possible significance for a novel approach to the therapy of inflammation. *Int J Tiss Res*, **VII**, 469-474

55.   Milanino, R, Conforti, A, Franco, L *et al*. (1985). Copper and inflammation - a possible rationale for the pharmacological manipulation of inflammatory disorders. *Agents and Actions*, **16**, 504-513

7
Copper therapy of inflammatory disorders: efficacy and biodistribution of topically applied copper complexes

SJ Beveridge
Department of Applied Sciences
Hunter Institute of Higher Education
PO Box 84 Waratah NSW 2298
Australia

I. INTRODUCTION

The use of copper devices, especially bracelets, for anti-inflammatory/anti-arthritic purposes goes back into folk-lore. Yet it is only of recent times that any serious attempt has been made to assess the validity or otherwise of the hypothesis that metallic copper can generate or promote anti-inflammatory activity *in vivo*. In providing some evidence for the probable therapeutic value of the copper bracelet, Walker and Keats[1] suggested that the components of sweat (especially amino acids) may act as cupriphores. Subsequently, the dissolution of copper in sweat was reported by Walker and Griffin[2]. Further evidence for the hypothesis was provided when Walker *et al.*[3] observed that ^{64}Cu-labelled bis(glycinato) copper(II) could permeate intact cat skin. In addition, the perfusion of human skin by copper(II) acetate has been reported by Odintsova[4]. Some evidence for the reactivity of metallic copper may be adduced from the observation that the crystalline solid bis(glycinato) copper(II) monohydrate can be isolated from an aerated aqueous solution of glycine containing metallic copper[5].

Because of the haphazard bioavailability of Cu(II) from the copper bracelet and the problems associated with other routes of administration, it was logical to ask: Why not use a topical application of pre-formed Cu(II)?

II. DEVELOPMENT OF A LIPOPHILIC COPPER SALICYLATE COMPLEX: ALCUSAL®

Although the therapeutic properties of salicylic acid have been known for

Copper and Zinc in Inflammation. Milanino, R, Rainsford, KD and Velo, GP (eds)
Inflammation and Drug Therapy Series, Volume IV

over a century[6], the suggestion that its mode of action may involve the chelation of a bioactive metal ion is comparatively recent. While Chenoweth[7] invoked chelation as relevant to the biological activity of salicylates, it was Schubert[8,9] who first suggested that salicylate delivered copper to the cells of the body and that a copper salicylate was involved in the anti-pyretic action of salicylates in rats. This suggestion essentially directs attention to the salicylate ion acting as a monodentate/bidentate ligand which facilitates tranfer of a key metal - such as copper(II) – to (or from) an inflammatory focus.

As $Cu(Hsal)_2.xH_2O$ (where Hsal = salicylic acid) complexes appeared to hydrolyse in aqueous solution forming 'basic mixtures', it was decided to work in non-aqueous media. This also had the advantage of emphasising the development of lipophilic compounds, which in themselves are more readily absorbed transdermally. The complex $Cu(Hsal)_2.EtOH$ was prepared by refluxing copper(II) hydroxide with salicylic acid in anhydrous ethanol[10]. Early preparations of Alcusal were formulated by dissolving the green crystalline complex (5.0 g) in an ethanol–glycerol mixture (1:1) (100 ml). These solutions had limited 'shelf-life', as an insoluble polymer was deposited. Reducing the amount of glycerol and increasing the concentration of free salicylic acid served to stabilise the complex in solution. Subsequent preparations of the solution avoided isolation of the free compound, while retaining the same concentration of the complex.

III. EFFICACY OF TOPICALLY APPLIED COPPER(II) FORMULATIONS

A number of bioassays were employed in determing the anti-inflammatory/anti-oedemic activity of a range of copper(II) formulations, including the copper(II) salicylate formulation described above.

In investigating the efficacy of the copper(II) salicylate preparation, a wide range of alternative potential cupriphores were also assessed. As part of this investigation, the copper(II) salicylate complex was prepared in a dimethyl sulphoxide (DMSO)–glycerol (4:1) solution (Dermcusal)[11]. The use of this solvent system also permitted comparisons between compounds which were of limited solubility in the ethanol–glycerol solvent described above. Irrespective of the bioassay employed, the protocol for topical application involved shaving an area of skin approximately 20 cm^2 on the dorsal surface of a rat, just below the neck[10].

1. Acute anti-inflammatory/anti-oedemic activity

Carrageenan, zymosan and hydroxylapatite–induced paw oedema were variously employed in determining the efficacy of the copper formulations, where the most effective showed the greatest inhibition of paw swelling. Significant loss in body weight of animals, during or immediately following the experiment, was used as a 'marker' of possible toxicity.

Because the experimental protocol called for exposing skin which was normally protected by hair, skin from the treated area was assessed for general condition and hair regrowth over a period of at least 4 days following the experiment.

The comparative activities of percutaneously applied copper(II) complexes in acute anti-inflammatory assays have been reported[10-12].

In summary[10,11], copper(II) salicylate proved effective in suppressing the acute inflammation associated with all the oedemogens indicated above. The paw inflammation triggered by microcrystalline hydroxylapatite is generally much less responsive to standard anti-inflammatory drugs than the corrageenan/yeast/kaolin oedemas. This inflammation was successfully controlled with the copper(II) salicylate formulation.

Maximum suppression of paw oedema was consistently observed when the oedema was initiated (by sub-plantar carrageenan injection) 6 hours after applying the ethanolic copper(II) salicylate preparation. There was no 'memory' of applying the preparation 24 hours previously. This is in distinct contrast to the 'memory' exhibited by more irritant Cu(II) formulations, such as copper(II) glycine administered subcutaneously: the anti-inflammatory effect being detectable up to 4 days thereafter.

In an attempt to draw some correlations between anti-inflammatory activity and ligand structure, some 30 copper(II) complexes were prepared[12], including phenols related to salicylic acid, metabolites of salicylic acid, short-chain fatty acids and a range of anti-inflammatory drugs. These included niflumic acid, phenylbutazone, diflunisal [5-(2,3-difluorophenyl) salicylic acid] and fenamole (1-phenyl-5-aminotetrazole).

From the results, a number of conclusions could be drawn.

(i) The presence of a 2-hydroxy group conferred useful drug activity, while a free carboxyl group was not essential for activity to be shown by copper complexes containing the 2-hydroxybenzoyl moiety.

(ii) Complexes involving the fatty acids exhibited little anti-inflammatory activity when compared to salicylic acid.

(iii) Percutaneously active copper(II) complexes were also formed with certain anti-inflammatory drugs, such as niflumic acid, phenylbutazone, that do not contain the hydroxybenzoyl moiety. When these drugs were applied alone (i.e. without the Cu(II)), they were much less effective than their respective copper complexes.

(iv) Topically applied Cu(I) complexes, prepared by reacting CuCl with various mercaptans (including 2-mercaptoethanol, N-acetylpenicillamine, D-penicillamine and 2-mercaptobenzoic acid) in DMSO, were uniformly devoid of anti-oedemic activity when assayed against carrageenan paw oedema.

2. Anti-arthritic activity

This was evaluated using an adjuvant-induced poly-arthritis. Rats developed overt signs of arthritis 12 days after inoculation with the adjuvant (delipidated *Mycobacterium tuberculosis* in squalane) into the tail near the base. At this time the thickness of the rear paws, the maximum width of the tail and the weight of animals were determined. An arbitrary score was assigned for inflammation in each front paw. Test formulations were applied daily for 4 days (either one or three times per day) and the above measurements repeated on day 16. The severity of the arthritis is reflected in the differences between these measurements.

Because the regime for drug application was over a substantially greater period of time than in the acute assays, the requirement to assess skin (for hair re-growth and general condition) which had been exposed to the topical application, was even more important. The anti-arthritic activity of dermally applied copper(II) salicylate and other copper(II) complexes has been reported[10-12]. From the results of these investigations, a number of significant points emerge.

(i)   Application of the ethanolic copper(II) salicylate complex (in ethanol-glycerol) to the shaved dorsal skin of rats suppressed development of further inflammatory signs in all four paws and tail with no adverse effect on body weight. At the conclusion of the experiment (day 16 from initial inoculation with adjuvant), the signs of inflammation increased in severity such that by day 20, the foot and paw swelling was as great as that of the control group at day 16. This 'rebound' phenomenon resembles that observed for perorally administered drugs, such as indomethacin and phenylbutazone, which only temporarily suppress signs of inflammation associated with severe polyarthritis.

(ii)   Of 28 copper(II) complexes which were tested against rats with established adjuvant-induced arthritis[12], only the copper complexes of phenylbutazone and niflumic acid were more potent than copper salicylate in DMSO. However, both these preparations caused more skin toxicity than the salicylate. While salicylic acid in DMSO shows little anti-arthritic activity, phenylbutazone and niflumic acid were moderately effective anti-arthritic drugs in this model.

IV. BIODISTRIBUTION OF COPPER IN RATS FOLLOWING TOPICAL APPLICATION

While data are available on the distribution and route of elimination following ingestion of copper salts[13], such data were lacking for dermally assimilated copper. Therefore the biodistribution of ^{64}Cu in various tissues, organs and excreta was investigated to assess (a) the extent of absorption and (b) the location and excretory pathway of radioactive copper internalised from the superficial dermis[14]. This study was subsequently extended to investigate the biodistribution of radioactive copper in inflamed rats[15]. This latter study was designed to identify ^{64}Cu-mobilisation in the rat in the presence of inflammation.

1. Biodistribution in normal rats

The experiments undertaken in this investigation[14] were designed to study transdermal uptake, biodistribution and route of elimination of the ^{64}Cu-labelled copper(II) salicylate complex in an ethanol–DMSO–glycerol (3:1:1) solvent.

The ^{64}Cu was extensively absorbed and excreted, primarily in faeces, after application of the lipophilic complex. Within 48 hours of applying the labelled copper salicylate complex, almost all of the ^{64}Cu had been cleared from the body. This accords with previous findings that the acute anti-inflammatory activity of ethanolic copper salicylate was of limited duration[10].

Topical application of a ^{64}Cu-labelled copper–phenylbutazone preparation revealed a similar pattern of ^{64}Cu biodistribution and excretion.

From this study it was concluded that copper(II) can pass rapidly through the dermal barriers when applied with an appropriate cupriphore and presented in a medium with low water content.

2. Biodistribution in inflamed rats

Two forms of inflammation were adopted in this study[15]. They were (i) a carrageen-induced acute paw oedema; and (ii) a chronic granulomatous response to an implanted irritant (heat-killed *Mycobacterium tuberculosis* in a polyurethane sponge).

Carrageenan was chosen as an acute inflammogen to determine whether any changes in ^{64}Cu biodistribution occurred due to a transient inflammatory stress. Overall, there was no difference between the inflamed and control groups in this acute model.

The longer-term, more chronic inflammation associated with the sponge granuloma significantly changed the biodistribution of endogenous copper. Following topical application of the ^{64}Cu-labelled copper(II) salicylate complex in ethanol–DMSO–glycerol (3:1:1) vehicle 5 days after implantation, total copper and radioactive copper levels were determined in the connective tissue capsule surrounding the sponge. The concentration of copper in this connective tissue was similar to that of the serum, reflecting a possible equilibrium. However, the activity of ^{64}Cu in this tissue indicated that *all* of the copper was probably due to copper from the labelled copper(II) salicylate formulation. This result suggested that copper moved to inflammatory sites and furthermore that the copper *in situ* was readily exchangeable. This was particularly apparent in the ^{64}Cu-salicylate treated

89

animals, where there was a relatively low level of ^{64}Cu in the serum, probably indicating targeting of this drug to inflammatory sites.

In addition, the concentration of copper in the sponge was higher than in the corresponding samples of blood or granulomae capsules. The high level of ^{64}Cu radioactivity found in the sponge indicates that exogenous ^{64}Cu – from the topically applied formulation – was sequestered at the inflammatory sites.

This may in part explain how copper complexes elicit their anti-inflammatory effect when administered percutaneously.

V. MODE OF ACTION

While the possible mechanisms of action for the anti-inflammatory/anti-arthritic activity of copper complexes are discussed elsewhere in this book, the properties of this unique copper(II) salicylate formulation and its mode of transfer warrant further comment.

In addressing the beneficial effects of topical copper(II) drugs, three hypotheses were proposed:

(i)   the copper-facilitated transfer of an anti-inflammatory ligand/ cupriphore across the normal dermal barriers; or

(ii)   local irritancy of the copper(II) within the dermis, rapidly eliciting an endogenous anti-inflammatory factor without necessarily requiring absorption of the copper into the bloodstream; or

(iii)   percutaneous absorption of copper(II) within the dermis, which then acts systemically.

The first hypotheses is unlikely to account for all the anti-inflammatory activity, as the levels of anti-inflammatory drugs attained by this mode of delivery are significantly below normal pharmacological levels[10].

The second hypothesis is unlikely, as data has been presented which shows that adrenalectomised animals still exhibit a rapid anti-inflammatory response[11].

Evidence adduced from the studies undertaken to date supports hypothesis (iii). In addition, the lack of toxicity associated with the ethanolic copper(II) salicylate is a significant feature. This may well arise because the co-tranferred salicylate not only reinforces the anti-inflammatory activity of the Cu(II) absorbed, but because it effectively minimises some of the commoner 'toxic' manifestations of applied Cu(II). In this novel complex, it would appear that there is a synergism, where the salicylic acid is co-transferring copper *and* the copper is co-transferring salicylic acid through the dermal barriers, providing a unique anti-inflammatory compound.

In a recent study, the ethanolic copper(II) salicylate complex was injected with the arthritogenic adjuvant. Following this injection, the normal progression of polyarthritis in the rats was suppressed. This activity is quite unlike any conventional anti-inflammatory drug (personal communication from M.W. Whitehouse).

VI. FUTURE DIRECTIONS

The majority of available studies which investigate the effect of copper in inflammation are based on assessment of total copper levels. It has become apparent however, that studies which adopt a protocol which permits some assessment of the *dynamic* changes in biodistribution of copper during inflammation provide a better understanding of the role of copper during inflammation. This approach will be extended to consider biodistribution of ^{64}Cu in rats with polyarthritis as well as changes which arise with administration of non-steroidal anti-inflammatory drugs.

ACKNOWLEDGEMENTS

An investigation into the biological roles of copper, especially in inflammatory disorders, led W. Ray Walker to pursue the successful development of a copper(II) salicylate anti-inflammatory formulation, suitable for topical application. I wish to acknowledge his insight in this field, which has produced significant developments and benefits.

Michael Whitehouse's investigative skills and long experience in the study of anti-inflammatory drugs has enabled the anti-inflammatory activities of copper drugs to be appreciated. The opportunity to collaborate with I. Ross Garrett in biodistribution studies has been greatly appreciated.

REFERENCES

1.   Walker, WR and Keats, DM (1976). An investigation of the therapeutic value of the Copper 'Bracelet'; Dermal assimilation of copper in arthritic/rheumatoid conditions *Agents Actions*, **6**, 454-459

2.   Walker, WR and Griffin, BJ (1976). The solubility of copper in human sweat. *Search*, **7**, 100-101

3.   Walker, WR, Reeves, RR, Brosnan, M and Coleman, GD (1977). Perfusion of intact skin by a saline solution of bis(glycinato) copper(II). *Bioinorg Chem*, **7**, 271-276

4.   Odintsova, NA (1978). Permeability of human skin to potassium and copper ions and their ultrastructural localization. *Chem Abs*, **89**, 360, Abs No 126707

5.   Beveridge, SJ and Walker, WR (1980). Formation of hydroxo-bridged copper(II) complexes by aeration of metallic copper. *Aust J Chem*, **33**, 2331-2335

6   Bekemeier, H (ed) (1977). *100 Years of the Salicylic Acid as an Anti-rheumatic Drug*, (Martin-Luther Universitat Halle-Wittenberg, Wissenschaftliche Beitrage), p.623

7.   Chenoweth, MB (1956). Chelation as a mechanism of pharmacological action. *Pharmocol Rev*, **8**, 57-87

8.   Schubert, J (1966). Chelation in medicine. *Sci Am*, **214**, (5), 40-50

9.   Schubert, J (1960). Chelation in medicine. In Seven, MJ and Johnson, LA (eds). *Metal Binding in Medicine*, (Philadelphia: Lippincott), p.325

10.   Walker, WR, Beveridge, SJ and Whitehouse, MW (1980). Anti-inflammatory activity of a dermally applied copper salicylate preparation (Alcusal®). *Agents Actions*, **10**, 38-47

11. Beveridge, SJ, Walker, WR and Whitehouse MW (1980). Anti-inflammatory activity of copper salicylates applied to rats percutaneously in dimethyl sulphoxide with glycerol. *J Pharm Phrmacol*, 32, 425-427

12. Beveridge, SJ, Whitehouse, MW and Walker, WR (1982). Lipophilic copper (II) formulations: some correlations between their composition and anti-inflammatory/anti-arthritic activity when applied to the skin of rats. *Agents Actions*, 12, 225-231

13. Bergqvist, U and Sundbom, M (1978). *Copper - Health and Hazard*. (Sweden: University of Stockholm Press)

14. Beveridge, SJ, Boettcher, B, Walker, WR and Whitehouse, MW (1984). Biodistribution of ^{64}Cu in rats after topical application of two lipophilic anti-inflammatory Cu(II) formulations. *Agents Actions*, 14, 291-295

15. Beveridge, SJ, Garrett, IR, Whitehouse, MW, Vernon-Roberts, B and Brooks, PM (1985). Biodistribution of ^{64}Cu in inflamed rats following administration of two anti-inflammatory copper complexes. *Agents Actions*, 17, 104-111

8

Concerning the chemistry and biology of some "copper-specific" ligands and their Cu complexes active as oral anti-inflammatory agents in the rat

M Bressan and A Morvillo
Dipartimento di Chimica Inorganica Metallorganica ed Analitica
Università di Padova
Centro CNR, Via Marzolo 1
35131 Padova, Italy, and
GP Velo*, E Concari*, U Moretti*, M Marrella* and R Milanino*
*Istituto di Farmacologia
Università di Verona
Policlinico Borgo Roma
37134 Verona, Italy

I. INTRODUCTION

As discussed elsewhere in detail[1,2], the rationale for the "copper approach" to the therapy of inflammatory disorders can be summarized as follows:

1.   The parenteral administration of copper compounds, can be considered to supplement copper that may sustain the natural response to inflammatory insult. It should be noted that the oral dosing appears to be often ineffective.

2.   The administration of ligands selective for copper and capable, at the same time, of forming stable complexes with the metal ("Cu-specific" ligands), can be considered to achieve manipulation of the endogenous copper ion *in vivo* to enhance its anti-inflammatory activity.

3.   The use of complexes of copper and "Cu-specific" ligands, might also be expected to overcome, at least in part, the problems concerned with the oral treatment.

The evaluation of the anti-inflammatory/anti-arthritic activity of various copper complexes including those formed with some classical non-steroidal anti-

Copper and Zinc in Inflammation. Milanino, R, Rainsford, KD and Velo, GP (eds)
Inflammation and Drug Therapy Series, Volume IV

inflammatory drugs has been the subject of previous extensive studies[3], whereas the investigation of the anti-inflammatory properties of both "Cu-specific" ligands, as suggested also by Jackson *et al.*[4], and their copper complexes, could be a promising novel approach, which, however, pose considerable challenges.

For example, a simple model for exploiting the delivery of endogenous copper, provides that the metal bound to plasma proteins is complexed by an administered "Cu-specific" ligand, copper-albumin being the most favourable target mainly because of its kinetic lability and pharmacological inactivity[5-8]. However, the low concentration of copper–albumin in the plasma (1 μM), its stability (log K_f = 16.2), and the fact that albumin itself is present in large molar excess in the blood (700 μM), would seem to lead to a requirement for strongly complexing agents in order to effectively mobilize significant quantities of copper into the low molecular weight fraction. In contrast however, the more powerful a chelating agent the more likely is to bind a variety of metals *in vivo* lacking selectivity. Moreover, such a strongly complexing agent should possess several powerful electron donor sites which are inclined to make the molecule polar, interfering with its ability to cross biological membranes. In fact EDTA is a good example of this situation. (For a comprehensive review of the above topics see also reference 9).

On the other hand, the oral administration of copper complexes, although formed with "Cu-specific" ligands, involves further problems, related to their instability in an environment of the gastric acidity. Oral administration of copper chelates which have been shown to possess anti-inflammatory activity when given parenterally, results in apparent lack of therapeutic effect. This lack of oral efficacy can be assumed to be due to the dissociation of the copper complexes in the upper gastrointestinal tract, with the consequence of a reduced copper absorption. The acidic environment in the stomach and duodenum is probably responsible for this dissociation[10-12]. In fact, in acidic media all basic donor groups of the ligands undergo some degree of protonation, resulting in the hydrogen ions being competitive with the metal ion (M^+) for the co-ordination by the donor groups of the ligand (L) [eq. 1], thus:

$$ML + H^+ \rightleftharpoons M^+ + HL \qquad [Eq. 1]$$

The co-ordinating properties of simple bases, like amines and carboxyl ions, are likely to be strongly affected by acidic media, and bases with low affinity for protons should then be favoured in order to make the metal complexes insensitive to changes in the pH. Unfortunately, the chemistry of copper(II) with this second class of donors (among which ethers, thioethers and phosphines are the most representative members) is rather poor and scarcely encouraging. In fact, ethers and (to a minor extent) thioethers yield only very unstable adducts[13,14], whereas phosphines usually promote fast reduction of copper(II) to copper(I) with oxidation of the ligands to phosphorus(V) derivatives[15].

II. CHOICE OF THE "Cu-SPECIFIC" LIGANDS

In view of the extreme complexity connected with the problems summarized above, and among the, nevertheless, almost countless approaches which could be employed to overcome these problems, we initiated a screening programme using the class of tridentate ligands outlined below, (Figure 7), which were found to produce stable 1:1 copper(II) adducts[16,17].

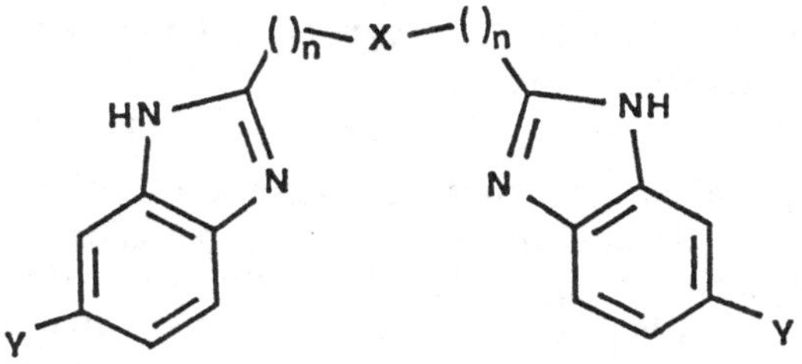

Figure 1 Tridentate ligands.
n = 1: Y = H, X = O(NON–C$_1$), X = S(NSN-C$_1$), X = NH(NNN–C$_1$)
  X = CH$_2$(NCN–C$_1$)
n = 2: Y = H, X = S(NSN), X = CH$_2$(NCN),
  Y = CH$_3$, X = S(NSN–Me)
  Y = Cl, X = S(NSN–Cl)

The rationale for this choice, employing the lead structure bis(2-benz-imidazoylyl)thioether (NSN), is summarized as follows.

1. The ligand contains imidazolyl and thioethereal groupings, which are found ubiquitously in a variety of biomolecules and also in the chemical environments of copper in many metalloproteins and enzymes.

2. The presence in the molecule of strongly-coordinating bases (e.g.. imidazole nitrogen atoms) may favour both a successful competition against endogenous complexes in biofluids, and the stability of the copper(II) adduct.

3. On the other hand, the presence in the molecule of a thioethereal sulphur donor may accomplish the following tasks.
   (i) It may give some degrees of selectivity with regard to commonly interfering cations, since R$_2$S groups are definitely poorer donors for "harder" (HSAB classification) ions (like Mg, Ca and Mn), compared with copper(II).
   (ii) It may favour the stability of the copper complex in acidic media, being different to that of the imidazole nitrogen atoms, a pH-insensitive donor.

95

III. CHEMISTRY OF NSN DERIVATIVES AND COPPER COMPLEXES

The lead NSN ligand yields stable copper(II) complexes, which have been isolated in the solid state, of the type $CuCl_2(NSN)$ and $Cu(ClO_4)_2(NSN)$. Also, the NSN ligand does not form complexes with calcium or magnesium, but does with zinc as $ZnCl_2(NSN)_2$. However, as expected from the Irving–Williams trend the copper complexes are more stable than those of zinc. Indeed, the water insoluble $ZnCl_2(NSN)_2$ adduct rapidly dissolves when in the presence of increasing amounts of $CuCl_2$, giving, quantitatively, coloured solutions of the $CuCl_2(NSN)$ species [eq. 2].

$$Zn(NSN_2^{2+} + 2\,Cu^{2+} \rightarrow 2\,Cu(NSN)^{2+} + Zn^{2+} \quad [eq. 2]$$

Competition experiments in aqueous solutions of $CuCl_2(NSN)$ with 20-fold excess of calcium, magnesium, zinc or manganese perchlorates have largely confirmed the remarkable higher stability of the copper(II) adduct. The UVV spectra, particularly those in the near-UV (320–340 nm), yield diagnostic absorption peaks, due to Ligand-to-Metal-Charge-Transfer (LMCT) $\sigma\,(S) \rightarrow d(Cu^{II})$ transition, which remain practically unchanged, once the necessary corrections for the intrinsic acidity of the different competing metal ions have been taken into consideration (Figure 2).

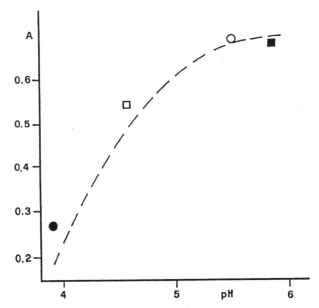

Figure 2 Absorbance (330 nm) of aqueous solutions of $CuCl_2$ (NSN).H_2O 2.45 mM, in the presence of $NaClO_4$ 1M. Dashed line = trend with pH (added HCl); solid squares = in the presence of $Mg(ClO_4)_2$ 50 mM (non buffered solution); open circles = in the presence of $Ca(ClO_4)_2$ 50 mM (non buffered solution); open squares = in the presence of $Zn(ClO_4)_2$ 50 mM (non buffered solution); solid circles = in the presence of $Mn(ClO_4)_2$ 50 mM (non buffered solution)

The copper(II) adducts with NSN, NSN–Cl and NSN–Me as ligands are extensively soluble in water (up to 5 mM) without apparent decomposition. Once dissolved, both copper chloride and perchlorate derivative adducts undergo rearrangement of the type ([eq. 3], in which X = Cl⁻ or ClO₄⁻):

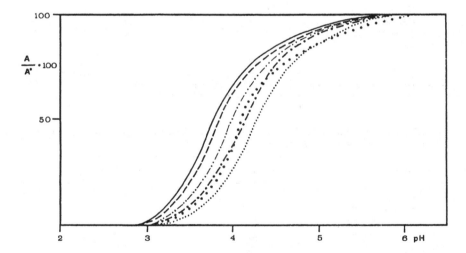

It should be noted that, particularly at lower concentrations and especially for the copper perchlorate derivatives, the 2:1 electrolyte (B in [eq. 3]) is the dominant species.

By addition of aq.HCl the copper complexes with the above NSN–Y ligands progressively collapse (Figure 3), but significant amounts of intact complexes are still present at definitely acidic pH values of about pH 3.0. Moreover, no negligible amounts (up to 10%) of copper(II) are still present in the complexed form, well over the addition of the stoichiometric quantities of HCl (i.e. 2 equivalents) required for the complete protonation of the ligands.

Figure 3 Fraction (molar %) of complexed copper(II) with pH (added HCl) for aqueous 1 mM solutions of different NSN–Y ligands. ———— = $CuCl_2(NSN)$; --------- = $CuCl_2(NSN-Cl)$; –·–·–·= $CuCl_2$ (NSN-Me); ***** = $Cu(ClO_4)_2(NSN)$; ········· = $Cu(ClO_4)_2(NSN-Cl)$;–··–··– = $Cu(ClO_4)_2(NSN-Me)$; A = actual adsorbance values of the 320–340 nm band; A° = adsorbance values of the 320–340 nm band at pH > 6.

Finally, with the exception of the adducts with the amino-group containing ligand (NNN–C$_1$), that dissolve in water, all other reported complexes are completely insoluble in water, where, by addition of HCl, progressively decompose without dissolving. Therefore, the "resistance" to HCl addition of these latter adducts, although measurable in some aprotic non-physiological solvent (e.g. ethanol or acetone), has not been taken into consideration in the present study.

IV. PHARMACOLOGY OF THE LIGANDS AND COMPLEXES

All the ligands synthesized (Figure 1) and their copper complexes prepared from either CuCl$_2$ or Cu(ClO$_4$)$_2$, were tested for acute anti-inflammatory activity in the carrageenan-induced paw oedema model in rats. The results obtained with the ligands alone, and with water soluble and insoluble complexes are shown in Table 1, 2 and 3 respectively.

Table 1   Anti-inflammatory activity in the carrageenan-induced paw-oedema test (CPO) of the rat:ligands

Compound		Number of rats	3 h CPO (% Inhib.)
1)	NSN	20	26**
2)	NSN–Cl	10	18
3)	NSN–Me	10	23**
4)	NCN	10	0
5)	NSN–C$_1$	15	2
6)	NNN–C$_1$	10	7
7)	NON–C$_1$	10	0
8)	NCN–C$_1$	10	8

All compounds were orally administered, 1 h prior carrageenan injection, at the dose of 0.32 mmol/kg.
** P < 0.01 (Student's t-test), versus vehicle-treated inflamed animals (N = 70 rats).
Details of the methods, and comparisons with different reference compounds are given in Reference 2.

Table 2   Anti-inflammatory activity in the carrageenan-induced paw-oedema test (CPO) of the rat: Cu complexes soluble in water

Compound		Number of rats	3 h CPO (% Inhib.)
9)	CuCl$_2$NSN	20	37**
10)	Cu(ClO$_4$)$_2$NSN	70	46**
11)	CuCl$_2$ NSN–Cl	10	28**
12)	Cu(ClO$_4$)$_2$ NSN–Cl	20	45**
13)	CuCl$_2$ NSN–Me	10	21*
14)	Cu(ClO$_4$)$_2$ NSN–Me	20	41**
15)	CuCl$_2$ NNN–C$_1$	10	0
16)	Cu(ClO$_4$)$_2$ NNN–C$_1$	10	0

All compounds were orally administered, 1 h prior carrageenan injection, at the dose of 0.32 mmol/kg.
* P < 0.05, ** P < 0.01 (Student's t-test), versus vehicle-treated inflamed animals (N = 70 rats).
Details of the methods, and comparisons with different reference compounds are given in Reference 2.

Table 3 Anti-inflammatory activity in the carrageenan-induced paw-oedema test (CPO) of the rat: Cu complexes insoluble in water

Compound		Number of rats	3 h CPO (% Inhib.)
17)	CuCl$_2$ NCN	10	0
18)	CuCl$_2$ NSN–C$_1$	15	11
19)	CuClO$_4$) NSN–C$_1$	15	0
20)	CuCl$_2$ NON–C$_1$	10	14
21)	Cu(ClO$_4$) NON–C$_1$	10	0
22)	CuCl$_2$ NCN–C$_1$	10	10
23)	Cu(ClO$_4$) NCN–C$_1$	10	10

All compounds were orally administered, 1 h prior carrageenan injection, at the dose of 0.32 mmol/kg. Statistic was made, using the Student's t-test, versus vehicle-treated inflamed animals (N = 70 rats). Details of the methods, and comparisons with different reference compounds are given in Reference 2.

In summary, the lead NSN ligand and its analogous NSN–Me showed some, though weak, anti-inflammatory activity (Table 1). The complexes soluble in water, with the sole exception of copper NNN–C$_1$ adducts, all showed oral anti-inflammatory activity, particularly when administered as perchlorate derivatives (Table 2). Finally, all those copper complexes insoluble in water were inactive as oral anti-inflammatory agents (Table 3).

After this initial approach, the most interesting molecules, i.e. the perchlorate derivatives of Cu–NSN–Y complexes (structures 10, 12 and 14, Table 2), and the NSN–Y ligands (structures 1, 2 and 3, Table 1), were further examined in acute and chronic animal models of inflammation. The results, which are reported elsewhere in detail[2], showed that one of the complexes, i.e. CuNSN (structure 10, Table 2), had:

(a)   dose-related anti-inflammatory activity when given orally in the acute carrageenan-induced paw oedema test of the rat[2], and

(b)   significant activity when administered orally, following a prophylactic regime, in the chronic adjuvant arthritis test in rats[2].

The above activities were both totally dependent upon the bioavailability, after oral administration, of some intact CuNSN complex into the gastrointestinal tract[2].

In view of the established "acid-resistance" of this complex,. we postulated that the oral administration of CuNSN could favour a greater inflow of copper within the inflamed organism, compared to that provided by the administration of CuCl$_2$. This hypothesis was initially tested by comparing the copper content of different key body compartments (i.e. plasma, liver, kidneys, and inflamed tissue), in acutely inflamed rats (carrageenan paw oedema), treated with equimolar amounts or oral CuCl$_2$, NSN, or CuNSN compared with that in control animals. Surprisingly, the results obtained (Table 4) contradicted the above theory, indicating that equal, and sometimes greater, amounts of copper are absorbed following a single oral admin-

Table 4 Paw-oedema weight and copper status in different body compartments, assessed 3 h after carrageenan injection (CPO) in orally-treated and control rats

Group	Paw oedema g (sd)	Plasma µg/ml(sd)	Liver Total µg(sd)	COPPER STATUS Kidneys Total µg(sd)	Infl. paw Total µg(sd)	Non-infl. paw Total µg(sd)
Absolute controls	--	1.39(0.04)	1.44(0.18)	34.80(1.93)	11.09(2.78)	1.31(0.06)**
Infl. vehicle-treated	1.01(0.15)	1.41(0.06)	1.40(0.21)	35.79(3.56)	11.95(2.23)	2.47(0.24)
Infl. CuCl2-treated	0.82(0.20)*	2.47(1.65)*	1.57(0.17)*	71.12(30.10)**	15.66(3.31)**	3.10(0.70)
Infl. NSN-treated	0.94(0.18)	1.53(0.32)	1.38(0.15)	36.14(4.44)	10.29(2.79)	2.52(0.27)
Infl. Cu(ClO4)2NSN-treated	0.59(0.13)**,+	2.10(0.31)**	1.49(0.22)	51.08(6.72)**	11.09(1.62)+	2.75(0.30)*

All substances were orally administered, 1 h prior carrageenan injection, suspended in 5% arabic gum, at the dose of 0.32 mmol/kg[2]. The rats were sacrificed 3 h after carrageenan injection: no statistically significant differences were observed comparing liver, kidneys and non-inflamed paw weights of any considered group. Copper determinations were done according to a previously published procedure[18].
Statistical analysis was made using the Student's t-test. N = 10 rats per group.
*P<0.05, ** P<0.01 comparison vs inflamed vehicle-treated group, + P<0.01 comparison vs inflamed CuCl2-treated group

istration of $CuCl_2$ than after CuNSN treatment, despite the latter showing significant inhibition of acute paw-inflammation (Table 4). Moreover, the ligand NSN alone, not only is virtually inactive as an anti-inflammatory agent, but also it does not appear to significantly modify, at least upon a single oral dosing, the copper status in the examined compartments.

V. CONCLUSIONS

The results obtained studying the chemistry and pharmacology of the ligands and copper complexes described in this paper, while preliminary, do allow some conclusions to be drawn, namely:

The ligands examined (NSN–Y in particular) have shown both selectivity for copper and capability of forming stable complexes with the metal *in vitro*. Nevertheless, the above chemical characteristics do not seem to have relevance *in vivo*, as the oral administration of these ligands failed to show a biologically significant anti-inflammatory activity, as well as to modify the status of copper in some key body compartments of acutely inflamed rats.

However, more encouraging results were found evaluating for anti-inflammatory activity, the copper(II) complexes of the above ligands. CuNSN deserves particular attention because of its appreciable pharmacological potential in both acute and chronic models of inflammation. The activity of this structure was shown to be dependent upon the presence of some intact copper(II) adduct in the gastrointestinal tract of administered rats[2]; yet, the preliminary results obtained studying the copper status in $CuCl_2$ and CuNSN treated animals, apparently indicate that, after oral administration, CuNSN is not capable of promoting a greater absorption of copper ions compared with $CuCl_2$. These observations raise questions concerning the mechanism of action of CuNSN in relation to its anti-inflammatory activity. Although the superoxide dismutase-like activity of Cu complexes could be the most favoured one[19], the mode of action of copper in the regulation of the inflammatory response is, however, not fully elucidated. As reviewed by Sorenson[3], other biochemical mechanisms (like the induction of lysyl oxidase, the modulation of prostaglandin synthesis, the stabilization of lysosomal membranes, etc.) may be invoked to account for the observed anti-inflammatory activity.

It goes without saying that the data and speculations summarized in this paper are essentially preliminary, and further experimental work is needed in order to draw safe conclusions. Nevertheless, the results are encouraging and do suggest a workable line to improve the effectiveness of these systems.

References

1. Milanino, R, Conforti, A, Franco, L, Marrella, M and Velo, GP (1985). Copper and inflammation – a possible rationale for the pharmacological manipulation of inflammatory disorders. *Agents Actions* 16, 504
2. Milanino, R, Concari, E, Conforti, A, Marrella, M, Moretti, U, Velo, GP, Rainsford,

KD and Bressan, M (1987). Synthesis and anti-inflammatory effects of some bis(2-benzimidazolyl) thioethers and their copper(II) chelates, orally administered in the rat. *Eur J Med Chem* (in press)

3. Sorenson, JRJ (1978). Copper complexes – a unique class of anti-arthritic drugs. In: Ellis, GP and West, GB (eds), *Progress in Medicinal Chemistry* Vol. 15, p. 211. (Amsterdam: Elsevier)

4. Jackson, GE, May, PM and Williams, DR (1978). Metal–ligand complexes involved in rheumatoid arthritis. VI. Computer models simulating the low molecular weight complexes present in blood plasma for normal and arthritic individuals. *J Inorg Nucl Chem* **40**, 1227

5. Laroche, MJ, Chappuis, P, Henry, Y and Rousselet, F (1982). Ceruloplasmin: experimental anti-inflammatory activity and physicochemical properties. In: Sorenson, JRJ (ed), *Inflammatory Diseases and Copper* p. 61. (Clifton, NJ: Humana Press)

6. Whitehouse, MW, Field, L, Ryall, RG and Denko, CW (1975). Is penicillamine a precursor drug? *Scand J Rheum* **4**, Suppl. 8, Abstr. 183

7. Brigelius, R, Spottl, R, Bors, W, Lengfelder, E, Saran, M and Weser, U (1974). Superoxide dismutase activity of low molecular weight Cu^{2+} chelates studied by pulse radiolysis. *FEBS Letters* **47**, 72

8. Brigelius, R, Hartmann, HJ, Bors, W, Saran, M, Lengfelder, E and Weser, U (1975). Superoxide dismutase activity of $Cu(Tyr)_2$ and Cu,Co-erythrocuprin. *Hoppe–Seyler's Z Physiol Chem* **356**, 739

9. May, PM and Bulman, RA (1983). The present status of chelating agents in medicine. In: Ellis, GP and West GB (eds), *Progress in Medicinal Chemistry* Vol. 20, p. 225. (Amsterdam: Elsevier)

10. Williams, DR, Furnival, C and May, PM (1982). Computer analysis of low molecular weight copper complexes in biofluids. In: Sorenson, JRJ (ed), *Inflammatory Diseases and Copper* p. 45. (Clifton, NJ: Humana Press)

11. Underwood, EJ (1977). Copper. In: *Trace Elements in Human and Animal Nutrition* 4th Edn., p. 56. (New York: Academic Press)

12. Perrin, DD and Whitehouse, MW (1981). Metal ion therapy: some fundamental considerations. In: Rainsford, KD *et al.* (eds), *Trace Elements in the Pathogenesis and Treatment of Inflammation* p. 261. (Basel: Birkhauser Verlag)

13. Sigel, H, Rheinberger, VM and Fischer, BE (1980). Stability of metal ion/alkyl thioether complexes in solution. Ligating properties of isolated sulfur atoms. *Inorg Chem* **18**, 3334

14. Bressan, M, Bon, ML and Marchiori, F (1982). Complexation of divalent metal ions with cyclo-L-methionyl-glycine in aqueous solution. *Inorg Chimica Acta* **67**, L47

15. Auliffe, MC and Levason, W (eds) (1979). *Phosphine, Arsine and Stibine Complexes of the Transition Elements* p. 201. (Amsterdam: Elsevier)

16. Dagdigian, JV and Reed, CA (1979). A new series of imidazole thioether chelating ligands for bioinorganic copper. *Inorg Chem* **18**, 2623

17. Amundsen, AR, Wheland, J and Bosnich, B (1977). Biological analogues. On the nature of the binding sites of copper-containing proteins. *J Am Chem Soc* **99**, 6730

18. Marella, M and Milanino, R (1986). Simple and reproducible method for acid extraction of copper and zinc from rat tissues for determination by flame atomic absorption spectroscopy. *Atomic Spectroscopy* **7**, 40

19. Deuschle, U and Weser, U (1985). Copper and inflammation. *Prog in Clin Biochem and Med* Vol. 2, p. 97. (Berlin: Springer-Verlag)

9
Zinc absorption and excretion in humans and animals

PE Johnson
United States Department of Agriculture
Agricultural Research Service
Grand Forks Human Nutrition Research Center
Grand Forks, North Dakota 58202, USA

I. INTRODUCTION

The existence of physiological controls on zinc metabolism may be inferred from the relatively small variations in tissue zinc levels which are observed in animals consuming diets varying widely in composition and zinc content.

Zinc metabolism is regulated by adjustments in both its absorption and excretion. This review will discuss the processes of zinc absorption and excretion and how they interact to achieve zinc homeostasis. Experimental data on the effects of specific foods or dietary components on the efficiency of zinc absorption will also be reviewed.

II. THE PROCESS OF ZINC ABSORPTION

1. Anatomical site of zinc absorption

Most research dealing with the site of zinc absorption along the intestine has been performed in the rat. Results have been conflicting, with some studies[1–5] suggesting that the duodenum is the major site of Zn absorption, while others[6] suggest that Zn absorption is fairly uniform along the length of the intestine or greater in the distal portion[7,8]. Thus Van Campen and Mitchell[1] injected Zn with a [65]Zn tracer into ligated segments of intestine, and measured uptake of the radioisotope into various tissues 3 h later. Zinc absorption occurred from the duodenum, jejunum, and ileum, respectively, in a ratio of about 7:1:3. In a similar experiment, Methfessel and Spencer[2] injected [65]Zn into ligated intestinal segments of non-fasted rats and found Zn was absorbed in a ratio of 2:1:1 from duodenum, jejunum, and ileum, respectively, after 2 h. Davies[3] injected a test dose of Zn with [65]Zn into the differ-

Copper and Zinc in Inflammation. Milanino, R, Rainsford, KD and Velo, GP (eds)
Inflammation and Drug Therapy Series, Volume IV

ent regions of the intestine, closed the surgical wound, and determined Zn absorption by measuring whole-body retention of ^{65}Zn over 8 days. This experiment showed Zn was absorbed in a ratio of 6:1:3 from the duodenum, jejunum, and ileum. Tissue uptake of ^{65}Zn 24 h after injection into various parts of the intestine in non-fasted rats showed greatest absorption from the duodenum and declining absorption along the length of the.intestine[4]. An early study[6] employed incubation of intact strips of intestine in a ^{65}Zn containing medium, showed approximately equal Zn absorption from the duodenum and ileum, with less absorption from the jejunum; however, no correction was made for differing total lengths of the different parts of the intestine. In contrast, Antonson et al.[7], using in vivo intestinal perfusion and a non-isotopic technique, found greater Zn absorption from the ileum (60%) than from the duodenum (19%) or jejunum (20%). They used non-fasted rats, and the total Zn dose in the perfusate was 200 μg, whereas other workers[1-3] used doses of 1 to 10 μg. These differences in experimental conditions might substantially affect results. Transfer of Zn from mucosa to serosa of everted sacs of intestine from rats, chickens, and hamsters was greater in the distal four-fifths of rat intestine than in duodenum, maximum in the distal ileum of chickens, but in hamsters was highest in the proximal duodenum[11]. Matseshe et al.[8] used a triple-lumen tube to measure intraluminal Zn at the ligament of Treitz and the proximal and distal jejunum after test meals in humans. They concluded that the site of Zn absorption was distal to the duodenum because more Zn passed the distal duodenum than was contained in any meal, and Zn disappeared from the two jejunal sites. The secretion of Zn into the duodenum does not, however, preclude the occurrence of Zn absorption in the duodenum.

The colon may play a minor part in the absorption of zinc. Sandström et al.[9] found ^{65}Zn absorption of 1–7% in human subjects after instillation of Zn into the colon. Davies[3] reported about 3% absorption from the colon in rats. A kinetic study of Zn absorption in adolescent rats[5] showed Michaelis–Menten kinetics with K_m values of 99, 45, and 50 μM and J_{max} values of 3.4, 2.7, and 1.2 μmol/h/g dry weight in proximal intestine, distal intestine, and colon, respectively. Adjusting for differing tissue weights, transport rates were 0.51, 0.37, and 0.20 μmol/h for proximal intestine, distal intestine, and colon, respectively. The role of the colon in Zn absorption may be affected by developmental changes. Net Zn absorption by adolescent rats in another study was approximately equal in jejunum, ileum, and colon, but absorption from the colon of suckling rats was four times greater than from jejunum or ileum[10].

Although the duodenum plays an important role in Zn absorption because of its faster rate of Zn transport than other parts of the intestine, it is apparent that the absorptive capacities of the rest of the small intestine, and the colon, are significant. Particularly when Zn doses are large, and because residence time of digesta is greater in the more distal part of the intestine[12], the ileum is probably the major site of Zn absorption.

2. Zinc absorption and transport into the circulation

There is some evidence that Zn absorption is an active process. Studies with the metabolic inhibitors 2,4-dinitrophenol and iodoacetate showed that mucosal to serosal Zn transport in everted intestinal sacs was reduced in their presence[11]. Incubation of tissue strips with 2,4-dinitrophenol did not result in reduction of tissue Zn uptake[6], but this method is probably less sensitive than the use of everted sacs.

Zinc absorption exhibits saturation kinetics when studied using a variety of experimental approaches[3,13–15]. This implies that zinc uptake across the brush border is a carrier-mediated process. Davies[3] measured Zn absorption from ligated intestinal loops *in vivo*, and found that Zn absorption was fairly linear for 15 min, and then declined. When the data were subjected to a double-reciprocal plot, a relationship characteristic of enzymic or carrier-mediated processes was observed. A K_m value of 2.1 mM and a J_{max} of 33 nmol Zn/min were obtained using doses up to 200 μg Zn. Zinc absorption measured in perfusion studies exhibited kinetics typical of a carrier-mediated process, with K_m values of 45 and 55 μM[5,13] and J_{max} values of 3–6 nmol/min[5,14]. Using isolated brush border membrane vesicles, Menard and Cousins[14] reported saturation kinetics with a K_m of 0.38 mM and J_{max} of 5.4 nmol/min/mg protein in vesicles from zinc-adequate rats and a K_m of 0.44 mM and J_{max} of 12 nmol/min/mg protein in vesicles from Zn-deficient rats. These data[14] and others[13] suggest that the brush border transport system for Zn is influenced by zinc status.

Kirchgessner and Weigand applied the Lineweaver–Burke treatment of data for Zn intake and true Zn absorption determined by isotope dilution in rats[15]. A double-reciprocal plot yielded a straight line and a Michaelis–Menten-type constant of 1.31 mg Zn/day, representing the Zn intake at half-maximum absorption rate. This intake corresponds to a dietary Zn level of about 115 ppm, far higher than the requirement for the growing rat, which is about 12 ppm[16,17]. This indicates that, under normal conditions, the capacity for zinc absorption is much greater than that which is observed, and that saturation of absorptive capacity would not be reached with a normal diet.

Saturation kinetics were observed in one perfusion study with mice[18], but not in another[19], which also failed to show a difference in the rate of Zn absorption between zinc-deficient and zinc-adequate mice. An intestinal perfusion study in humans failed to show Michaelis–Menten kinetics. Zn absorption was linearly related to its intraluminal concentration over a range 0.1–0.9 mM Zn in the perfusion solution[20]. This probably approximates intestinal concentrations after meals containing moderate or high amounts of Zn[8]. However, that study[20] did show that glucose and glycyl-leucine, but not glycine + leucine, enhanced Zn absorption, which implied a possibility of carrier-mediated transport in humans despite the fact that saturation kinetics were not observed.

Carrier-mediated transport is not fully developed in the suckling rat[5];

saturation kinetics were reported in the proximal intestine of suckling rats, the proximal and distal intestines of weanling rats, and in the proximal and distal small intestine and colon of adolescent rats.

The nature of the carrier is not known. However, in zinc-deficient rats, brush-border proteins of approximately 43,000 and 63,000 daltons were more abundant than in zinc-adequate rats[21]. Wapnir and Stiel[22] recently investigated structural characteristics of ligands which enhance Zn uptake at the brush border in an effort to characterize the mechanism involved in Zn uptake. They found that Zn absorption was greater in the presence of amino acids than of amino acid homologues. Amino acids were involved in both mediated and non-mediated Zn transport, but only non-mediated Zn uptake was observed in the presence of homologues.

3. Effect of solutes in the lumen

Intestinal secretions and the digesta contain a variety of organic molecules, such as amino acids, which have the potential to chelate zinc and to enhance or inhibit its absorption. Many of these molecules originate from the digestion of food, and their effects will be described in the section on zinc absorption from foods. There have also been proposals that certain small molecules of physiological origin might not only enhance zinc absorption, but, indeed, be required.

Hahn and Evans[23] first reported the association of zinc with a low molecular weight ligand in the intestinal lumen and mucosa of rats after an oral dose of ^{65}Zn. Evans et al.[24] reported that this ligand was of pancreatic origin in rats and dogs, and that zinc absorption was markedly decreased in rats after ligature of the common bile duct. Zinc absorption was restored to normal when zinc was administered orally with a pancreatic extract to animals that had ligated common bile ducts[24]. Subsequently, various investigators reported this zinc-binding ligand (ZBL) to be amino acid residues[25,26], N,N,N'-trimethylaminediamine[27], prostaglandin E_2 [28,29], and picolinic acid[30]. The report of N,N,N'-trimethylaminediamine was shown to be an artefact of the purification procedure used[31]. Cousins et al.[32] showed that the amino acid residues and the ZBL might be breakdown products of metallothionein.

Prostaglandin E_2 increased mucosal-to-serosal zinc absorption by everted jejunal sacs[29,33], whereas $PGF_{2\alpha}$ had the opposite effect. Oral administration of PGE_2 to rats increased the ^{65}Zn content of internal organs[33]. Evans reported PGE_2 in the ZBL-containing fraction of porcine duodenum[28] and found that when rats were fed [^{14}C]arachidonic acid, a precursor of PGE_2, the ^{14}C and ^{65}Zn appeared in identical fractions, which reacted to PGE_2 antibodies. In addition, administration of aspirin, an inhibitor of PGE_2 synthesis, inhibited ^{65}Zn absorption in rats. However, many investigators believe prostaglandins to be unimportant in normal zinc absorption, since oxygen-rich molecules are poor binders of zinc[34], and prostaglandins are present in tissues in concentrations much lower than that of zinc. Most experiments reported have been with very high levels of the prostaglandins. However, these findings suggest that a role for prostaglandins in Zn absorption should not be overlooked.

Picolinic acid, a tryptophan metabolite, enhances zinc absorption under certain conditions. Seal and Heaton[35] reported that picolinic acid increased the uptake of zinc by everted intestinal sacs. When they fed rats 50 ppm dietary Zn and a 50-fold excess of picolinic acid, turnover of ^{65}Zn was accelerated[36]. Two studies[37,38] employed intestinal perfusion techniques in rats that had been fed diets with about 58 ppm Zn. Wapnir[37] found that PA:Zn ratios greater than 3:1 (approx. 450 μM PA) adversely affected the rate of zinc absorption, and that picolinic acid was less effective than most other ligands tested in promoting zinc absorption, but he made no comparison to a perfusate containing no ligand. Oestreicher and Cousins[38] found no difference in the rate of zinc absorption from perfusion solutions with a 17:1 PA:Zn ratio (110 μM PA) and a control solution containing no ligand. Jackson[39] fed rats 30 ppm Zn and gavaged them with a solution of ^{65}Zn and picolinic acid having a PA:Zn ratio of 2.8. After 4 h, no increase in Zn absorption was seen compared to rats given ZnCl$_2$ alone. However, when rats were fed a tryptophan-limiting diet containing 8 ppm Zn, the addition of picolinic acid to the diet increased zinc absorption from 59% to 98%[40,41]. The addition of picolinic acid to a 20% zein + lysine diet increased zinc absorption from 59% to 98%[40,41]. In a study with men fed a tryptophan-limiting diet and 2.9 mg Zn/d, addition of 10 mg picolinic acid/d to the diet resulted in a significant increase in zinc absorption (Johnson, PE *et al.*, unpublished). In general, picolinic acid does not seem to affect zinc absorption and metabolism when given in a single oral dose or perfusate, but only when fed on a chronic basis as part of the diet. Its effects are most pronounced when the zinc content of the diet is marginal.

Recently Wapnir and Stiel[22] investigated structural characteristics that might be required for ligands to enhance zinc absorption. They observed both mediated and non-mediated transport mechanisms for amino acids, but only non-mediated zinc uptake for amino acid homologues. Blocking or deletion of either the carboxyl group or the amino or the imino group of amino acids seemed to interfere with Zn absorption. The effect was much less when the homologue itself was a good chelator (i.e. imidazole).

A low molecular weight ligand similar to that in intestine was observed in human milk[30,42–44]. Evans and Johnson reported that it was picolinic acid[45], while other investigators identified it as citrate[46–48]. The identity of the ligand in human milk was of interest because of the efficacy of human milk in treatment of acrodermatitis enteropathica[49], a genetic zinc-deficiency disease[49] in which a defect in zinc absorption has been reported[50–52]. It was postulated that the ZBL was absent or low in neonatal rat intestine, but present in the intestines of older rats[44,53]. Thus the ZBL might be necessary for Zn absorption during the neonatal period. Both picolinic acid and citrate have been reported to enhance or have no effect on Zn absorption[35–41] and picolinic acid has been reported to be efficacious in the treatment of acrodermatitis enteropathica[54]. There was considerable controversy over the identity of 'the' zinc-binding ligand in human milk and its role in normal zinc absorption[55–60]. Apparently this was a case of not seeing the forest for the trees. Neither citrate nor picolinic acid account completely for the reported differences in zinc absorption[61–63] from human milk and cow's milk or infant formulas. Most likely both of these small molecules and others, as well as peptides or small proteins in milk, are responsible for observed differences in zinc absorption from human milk and other milks. Further investigations of the effects of both citrate and picolinic acid on zinc metabolism are warranted.

4. Intracellular events

Considerable efforts have been made to elucidate the nature of the protein(s) or other ligands within the intestinal cell which are responsible for the absorption of zinc across the cell membrane and its transfer through the cell[64–67]. This remains an area where only a general outline of the process is known.

Starcher[68] first showed in 1969 that Zn could displace ^{64}Cu from a protein of approximately 10,000 daltons in the duodenal mucosa of chicks. Evans[69] found that Zn could displace Cu from metallothionein in bovine duodenum. Subsequently, Van Campen and Kowalski[70] and Kowarski et al.[11] reported that ^{65}Zn in rat intestinal mucosa was bound mostly to a high molecular weight (HMW) fraction of about 10^5 daltons, as well as to a medium-weight fraction (MMW) of 10,000–12,500 daltons. The MMW fraction was purified and identified as metallothionein by Richards and Cousins[71].

Synthesis of metallothionein can be induced by feeding or injection of Zn[64,71–75]. This finding led Cousins to propose that intestinal Zn absorption was regulated by the induction of metallothionein[66,75,76]. He suggested that excess Zn induced metallothionein synthesis; this metallothionein would bind Zn in intestinal cells. However, synthesis of metallothionein is induced only by large amounts of Zn[75,77], and maximum response is observed 5–6 h after the inducing Zn dose, although absorption takes place much more quickly[19]. Brief exposure to zinc did not increase intestinal metallothionein levels in mice[78]. Thus, although metallothionein may be involved in relatively long-term modulation of Zn status, through involvement in zinc excretion, metallothionein's resistance to induction by normal levels of dietary Zn suggests that it is probably not a zinc carrier molecule for the process of absorption. Metallothionein may function as a rapidly turned-over storage protein[78], or as a buffering agent for Zn moving between HMW and LMW ligands[79]. Coppen and Davies[80] found that when dietary Zn varied between 20 and 160 mg/kg, the biological half-life of body Zn stores appeared to be inversely related to the metallothionein content of the duodenum. The regulation of zinc absorption by metallothionein would not account for the separate effects of Zn status and Zn dose in a meal on percentage Zn absorption[80,81]. The reciprocal relationship between metallothionein and Zn, which is central to Cousin's hypothesis, was not observed in mice[19].

Intracellular proteins other than metallothionein are involved in zinc absorption, but their roles are not well defined. Kowarski et al.[11] found more of a HMW protein (about 10^5 daltons) in homogenates of jejunal mucosa than in duodenal mucosa. This corresponded to a higher rate of zinc transport in the jejunum than in the duodenum. Zinc-deficient rats had relatively more Zn bound to a HMW ligand than rats fed a normal diet[79]. Chromatography of duodenal mucosa cytosol on Sephadex G-75 showed reduced incorporation of ^{65}Zn into a HMW band of 55,000 daltons when KCN and NaF were added to the incubation mixture[82]. Thus, transfer of Zn to the HMW protein may be an active process.

III. ZINC HOMEOSTASIS

The existence of controls on Zn metabolism can be inferred from the fact that tissue and whole-body levels of Zn are nearly invariant within a wide range of intakes above the requirement. Pallauf and Kirchgessner[83] fed rats diets containing from 2.2 to 500 mg Zn/kg, and found that whole-body Zn was constant between intakes of 15 and 100 mg/kg and that bone zinc did not change between intakes of 20 and 100 mg Zn/kg. Below intakes of 15 mg Zn/kg and at 500 mg/kg, bone and whole-body Zn were related to Zn intake. Deeming and Weber[84] also found little change in bone or plasma Zn when rats were fed diets with 12 or 68 mg Zn/kg, but values were lower when diets contained 3 or 6 mg Zn/kg. Cotzias first showed that zinc homeostasis is controlled by variations in both the absorption and the turnover of zinc[85]. He found that turnover of ^{65}Zn was accelerated by administration of a zinc salt, and that zinc absorption decreased when an intraperitoneal Zn load was given before the oral dose. Subsequently, many investigators reported a generally inverse relationship between dietary Zn and Zn absorption in rodents[13,14,39,80,81,86–92], ruminants[93,94], and humans[95,96] and increased excretion or turnover of Zn with increased dietary Zn[89–91,93,94,97,98]. A decrease in percentage absorption with increasing dose in a meal has also been noted in rodents[19,39,80,81] and humans[95,99].

Coppen and Davies[80] found that percent absorption (y) of an oral dose of ^{65}Zn was inversely related to dietary Zn (x) in an exponential fashion, such that

$$y = 4.488x^{(-0.73)}, r^2 = 0.96.$$

They found a similar relationship between biological half-life ($T_{1/2}$) of Zn (y) in hours and dietary Zn (x):

$$y = 135.5x^{(-0.18)}, r^2 = 0.95.$$

Thus, as dietary Zn increased, the absorption decreased and rate of turnover of Zn increased (biological half-life decreased). Zn absorption changed most rapidly at low dietary Zn levels, while the biological half-life changed more rapidly at higher levels of dietary Zn.

Weigand and Kirchgessner, using an elegant isotope dilution technique[100], have studied the dependence of endogenous faecal Zn excretion on dietary intake. They reported that, in rats, when dietary Zn was below the requirement, faecal Zn was entirely of endogenous origin[89–91]. Under these conditions zinc absorption was close to 100%. As dietary zinc increased above the requirement, percentage absorption decreased, and the amount of endogenous faecal excretion increased. Urinary Zn was slightly lower in zinc-deficient rats, but varied little with dietary zinc intakes above the requirement. They interpreted these data as showing that when dietary zinc is much greater than the requirement, homeostatic control is exerted through variations in absorption, and when dietary Zn is near the requirement, control is exerted through changes in endogenous faecal excretion. When dietary Zn was 18.2 mg/kg, 93.3% of intake was absorbed, and endogenous faecal excretion was 25.5 μg/d[90]. When dietary Zn was 10.6 mg/kg, 97.6% of intake was absorbed, and endogenous excretion was only 6.3 μg/d. Thus, changes in endogenous faecal Zn excretion played the primary role in regulation when Zn intake was near the requirement, although even at that level of Zn intake, percentage absorption changed with the dietary supply. When dietary Zn varied from 39 to 141 mg/kg, a 3.6-fold change, Zn absorption decreased and endogenous faecal excretion increased, both by a factor of about 2.5. Therefore, Weigand and Kirchgessner's conclusion that homeostatic control was exerted by changes in absorption at high Zn intake was only partially correct, because absorption and endogenous excretion varied in tandem.

Evans et al.[92] likewise proposed that Zn metabolism was regulated by Zn excretion into the intestine, and that reports by previous investigators showing decreases in percent Zn absorption with increasing intake were caused by dilution of orally administered isotope by endogenous Zn secretion into the intestine. This argument is partially true, and substantiated by the marked difference in absorption values between rats given oral and intramuscular ^{65}Zn that Evans observed. However, when the isotope dilution technique was used to correct for endogenous Zn, Evans still observed a fall in percentage Zn absorption from 91% to 71% when intake was increased from 169 μg/d to 275 μg/d. It can be calculated from his data that endogenous faecal Zn increased about 3-fold at the same time.

Data obtained in my laboratory support the concept that Zn absorption and excretion vary in tandem to control Zn metabolism, but suggest that the controls on these two functions may differ. An experiment was done to examine the effect of past diet or body Zn stores and current diet on Zn absorption and endogenous excretion[101]. Rats were fed diets containing 1.5, 12, or 50 mg Zn/kg for 19 days ('past diet'), and switched to diets containing 3, 12, 20 or 50 mg Zn/kg ('present diet'). Zn absorption, endogenous excretion, and balance were measured using an isotope dilution technique after 21 days of the second dietary period. The results of this experiment are shown in Table 1. Percent absorption of Zn was affected only by the present diet, but endogenous excretion was affected by both the past and present diet.

Table 1   Zn balance, absorption and endogenous excretion

Group	Dietary Zn (mg/kg) First period	Second period	Urine excretion (μg/d)	Balance (μg/d)	Endog- enous faecal excretion (μg/d)	Zn absorp- tion (%)
A I	1.54	3.65	1	31	6	88.2
II		12.64	4	121	46	78.6
III		20.46	6	111	92	63.6
IV		50.32	7	112	173	33.9
B I	12.64	3.65	3	33	11	89.2
II		12.64	8	81	64	73.0
III		20.46	7	76	121	62.8
IV		50.32	8	48	224	33.5
C I	50.32	3.65	1	35	13	92.8
II		12.69	5	77	73	74.8
III		20.46	9	61	113	51.9
IV		50.32	6	75	217	33.9
Root MSE			4	52	19	9.6
ANOVA Past diet (A–C)			NS	(0.06)	0.0001*	NS
Present Diet (I–IV)			0.0001	0.0068	0.0001	0.0001
Past x present		NS	NS	NS	NS

*By Scheffe contrasts, Group A is significantly different from groups B and C (p = 0.0001), but B and C do not differ.

The past diet significantly decreased endogenous fecal Zn only in the group which was fed a Zn-deficient diet during the first period. Furthermore, total-body Zn and tissue Zn concentrations were decreased at the end of the first dietary period in rats fed 1.5 mg Zn/kg, but groups fed 12 or 50 mg Zn/kg did not differ. By the end of the second dietary period this difference in tissue Zn concentration in rats fed 1.5 mg Zn/kg in the past diet had been mostly made up, so that values in rats fed 1.5 mg Zn/kg in the past diet were similar to those in rats fed 12 or 50 mg Zn/kg in the past diet. Because percentage Zn absorption from the present diet was not affected by the past diet, this catch-up in tissue Zn concentration had to have been caused by alterations in endogenous Zn excretion. These data show that both Zn absorption and

111

endogenous excretion are responsive to dietary Zn intake. In addition, there is some internal mechanism for regulating excretion of Zn which responds to the tissue Zn levels; by this means the body attempts to maintain tissue Zn at a particular level.

Kinetic analysis of zinc metabolism in normal humans, using [65]Zn, identified five sites of regulation of zinc metabolism[102]. Tissue zinc concentrations were regulated by absorption of zinc from gut, excretion of zinc in urine, secretion of zinc into gut, release of zinc by muscle, and exchange of zinc with erythrocytes[102].

Other avenues of potential Zn losses are hair, sweat, menses, semen, and milk. While the amount of Zn lost by these routes is usually small compared to faecal losses, there is evidence that they are also subject to some homeostatic control. Most milk Zn comes directly from the mother's dietary intake during lactation, and only about 10% from body Zn stores[103]. When dairy cows or rats were fed diets low in Zn there was a corresponding decrease in milk Zn[104–106]. Diets very high in Zn (1000–2000 mg/kg) resulted in increased milk Zn in cows[107]; however, within the range of normal dietary intakes, dietary Zn was unrelated to milk Zn in women[108,109] and supplements of 20–60 mg Zn/d failed to increase milk Zn[110–112]. When men were fed diets containing only 3.6 mg Zn/d, zinc losses in sweat declined gradually with time[113]. When diets contained 33.7, 8.3, and 3.6 mg Zn/d, average sweat Zn losses were 0.62, 0.49, and 0.24 mg/d, respectively, suggesting that there is some homeostatic control of sweat Zn. Others have reported similar reductions in sweat Zn with decreased Zn intake[114]. The amount of Zn in hair or wool of animals has been shown to be related to the Zn content of the diet[115,116]. In humans, no correlation was observed between hair Zn and either plasma or red cell Zn for a population consuming self-selected diets[117], but exposure to high levels of Zn in an industrial setting (galvanizing) resulted in increased hair and toe-nail Zn[118]. Zinc loss in menses[119–121] is approximately 0.2–0.4 mg/d. It is not known if this varies with dietary Zn. Zinc in semen is in the range of 0.01 to 0.6 mg/ml, or 0.08 to 1.7 mg Zn per ejaculum[122–125]. Seminal zinc levels fell in men fed 0.3 mg Zn/day for 4–9 weeks[125].

IV. ZINC ABSORPTION FROM FOODS AND FOOD COMPONENTS

1. Physiological factors affecting absorption

Although animal studies of Zn absorption have tended to employ male weanling or adolescent rats, it is important to note that age, sex, growth, pregnancy, and disease can all affect zinc absorption, albeit to different degrees. Aamodt *et al.* reported that mean absorption of Zn decreased linearly with age, by about a tenth of a per cent per year, over an age range of approximately 20 to 75 years of age[126]. This decrease, though small, was highly significant ($r = -0.934, p < 0.001$). Absorption decreased more rapidly with age in women than in men, but women absorbed more zinc than men in all but one age category. This difference was also significant when subjects were compared by decade using a paired t-test. Turnlund and co-workers[127,128] found lower absorption ($17 \pm 3\%$) in men aged 65–74 than in young men ($25 \pm 6\%$) aged 21–33 on diets containing 15–16.5 mg Zn/d.

In rats, zinc absorption was greater in suckling animals than in adolescents[5,10]. This is probably because intestinal permeability is greater in the suckling than in the more mature animal. Using isolated everted intestinal sacs, Schwarz et al. found that Zn absorption increased during pregnancy in the rat[129] until, during the third trimester, it was significantly higher than in non-pregnant, non-lactating controls. Absorption of zinc remained higher during the first few days of lactation, and then fell to control levels. Using a stable isotope of Zn, Swanson et al. measured Zn absorption in pregnant and non-pregnant women, but found no increase in Zn absorption during pregnancy[130] when women at approximately 30 weeks gestation were fed a diet containing about 17 mg Zn/d. It seems possible, however, that changes in zinc absorption during pregnancy might be measurable under conditions of less adequate dietary intake, or if longitudinal rather than cross-sectional measurements could be made.

Various diseases have also been shown to affect zinc absorption and excretion. Absorption of zinc is decreased in alcoholism[131], Crohn's disease[132], inflammatory bowel disease[133], pancreatic insufficiency[134], anorexia nervosa[135], and acrodermatitis enteropathica[136,137]. In cattle with Adema disease, an inherited trait similar to acrodermatitis enteropathica, zinc absorption is impaired[138,139]. Mucosal zinc uptake is lower in diabetic rats[140], because of mucosal hyperplasia, but changes in zinc absorption in diabetic humans have not been reported. Urinary excretion of zinc is increased in cirrhosis[141], and massive losses of zinc occur in patients with severe burns[141]. Whole-body loss of zinc was several times greater than normal in man with gluten enteropathy, although absorption of zinc was normal (GI Lykken and PE Johnson, unpublished data).

2. Methodological considerations

The balance method has been the classical means of assessing zinc absorption in humans. However, because endogenous excretion via the faeces, as well as absorption, can be affected by diet, it should be clear that zinc balance does not give an accurate indication of zinc absorption. Balance measurements are useful because they show the net effect of both absorption and excretion, but they do not provide any mechanistic information. Techniques for measurement of zinc absorption will be discussed briefly here, because not all techniques yield the same kind of information.

(a)   Whole-body retention of zinc following a radioisotope dose

Heth and Hoekstra[142] developed the now classic method for determining zinc absorption using radioactive zinc. Briefly, animals are dosed orally with radioactive zinc, and whole-body retention of the isotope is monitored for a period of days or weeks. Another group of animals receiving a similar diet is injected with the isotope and its retention determined. When a semi-log plot of percentage retention versus time is made, the curve becomes linear after 3–5 days. The linear portions of these plots are extrapolated to the time of dose, and true absorption is defined as the intercept of the oral retention plot divided by the intercept of the injected retention plot. The data from the animals who received the isotope by injection are thus used to correct for endogenous excretion of zinc. The slope of the semi-log plot gives an indication of zinc turnover, and biological half-life can be calculated from the slope.

This approach is often used without a group receiving the isotope by injection, when test meals differing from the basal diet are fed. In such cases apparent absorption rather than true absorption is determined, but relative differences among test meals are assumed to be the same as if the correction for endogenous excretion had been made. Use of radioisotopes of zinc to measure apparent absorption in this way has been extremely useful in human studies[143,144]. The kinetics of zinc excretion have also been investigated using whole-body measurements of ^{65}Zn or ^{69m}Zn retention[98,102,145–150].

(b)   Dual isotope faecal collection procedure

Payton et al.[151] have described a rapid method for measuring zinc absorption in humans without the necessity for a whole-body gamma counter or prolonged periods of observation. It involves the simultaneous administration of ^{65}Zn and ^{51}Cr, and the measurement of the ratio of the two isotopes in a single faecal sample. The ^{51}Cr serves as an inert, non-absorbable marker. This method may be confounded by the administration of lactulose to promote defaecation as soon as possible after the ^{65}Zn dose, thus shortening the residence time of zinc in the gastrointestinal tract. It gives the same results as whole-body retention measurements of zinc absorption in subjects who are also given lactulose.

(c)   Faecal monitoring of stable isotopes of zinc

Naturally occurring zinc is composed of five stable (non-radioactive) isotopes: ^{64}Zn, 48.89%; ^{66}Zn, 27.81%; ^{67}Zn, 4.11%; ^{68}Zn, 18.56%; ^{70}Zn, 0.62%. If one of these isotopes is administered orally, the unabsorbed portion appears in the faeces, and the isotopic composition of the faeces differs from normal. Absorption is calculated as the difference between the oral isotope dose and the faecal isotope in excess of the natural abundance. The isotopes which are naturally least abundant are the best 'tracers', because a small dose of highly enriched isotope will produce a fairly large change in the isotopic abundance ratios. The least abundant isotopes are the most expensive, so that methodological concerns usually must be balanced by financial considerations. Faecal monitoring does not give a completely accurate measurement of absorption because some excretion of absorbed isotope occurs during the week or two that is required for faecal collection. For zinc, this is about 10% of the isotope dose[145]. Thus, values obtained by faecal monitoring are best referred to as apparent absorption. Another factor which may affect interpretation of data is that doses on the order of a few milligrams of isotope must be used, so that this is not a tracer method in the usual sense.

Isotopic analysis of faeces or other samples can be done by two basic techniques: neutron activation analysis[152–154] or mass spectrometry (MS). Only three of the stable isotopes of zinc, ^{64}Zn, ^{66}Zn, and ^{70}Zn, can be analysed by neutron activation analysis. Mass spectrometric methods which can be used include direct probe-MS of metal chelates[155] or gas chromatography-MS of metal chelates[156], fast atom bombardment–MS[157], and thermal ionization–MS[158–160]. Of these methods, thermal ionization is the most precise and the slowest. In comparisons of thermal ionization-MS and neutron activation analysis, thermal ionization-MS was found to give superior results[154]. Comparisons of absorption determined by faecal monitoring using stable isotopes or radioisotopes have been made in humans[158] and rats[161] and there was no difference in absorption values with the method of analysis. Stable isotopes have also been used for kinetic studies of zinc in blood[162].

(d) Isotope dilution

An isotope dilution technique for measuring both true absorption and endogenous excretion of zinc was developed by Weigand and Kirchgessner[100]. Animals are injected with radioactive zinc, and after a period of equilibrium (about 9 days), faeces are collected and food intake measured. At the end of the balance period the specific activity of blood or tissue is determined and compared to the specific activity of faeces. Absorption is calculated as:

$$A = \frac{I\,F + S_f/S_m(F)}{I}$$

where A is fractional absorption, I is intake, F is faecal Zn, S_f is specific activity of faeces, S_m is specific activity of tissues. The term $S_f/S_m(F)$ represents the endogenous faecal excretion. This method has the advantage of determining Zn absorption from the *ad libitum* diet over a period of several days, and may provide a more accurate indication of absorption than methods which employ a single test meal.

Jackson et al.[163] adapted this method to employ intravenous infusion of a stable zinc isotope in human subjects.

115

(e) Plasma tolerance curves

Several investigators have measured changes in plasma zinc after an oral zinc dose[134,164–169], reasoning that increases in plasma zinc must be directly related to the zinc most recently absorbed. This method is attractive because sample collection is complete in about 4 h, and only blood need be collected. This makes it useful for field studies. However, most studies have used doses of 25 mg or even 50 mg of elemental Zn. Use of these pharmacological doses may result in findings which are not necessarily the same as would be obtained with more normal Zn doses. Ingestion of meals which are not supplemented with Zn often results in a decrease in postprandial Zn, rather than an increase[170]. Changes in postprandial Zn may reflect differences in rates of Zn absorption rather than in total Zn absorption[171].

(f) Slope-ratio assays: growth or bone Zn response

Differences in growth or incorporation of Zn into bone have been used to assess Zn bioavailability in animals. Such methods necessarily employ young growing animals that are fed suboptimal levels of Zn. Different concentrations of dietary levels of Zn are achieved by incorporating different levels of the test substance into the diet as the Zn source. Response to the different amounts of the Zn source is compared to response to graded amounts of a Zn salt. Growth is a particularly non-specific criterion, because the diets which contain different amounts of Zn also contain different amounts of all the components, nutritive and otherwise, which are in the test food. Bone Zn concentrations in rats are not correlated with dietary Zn above 12 mg/kg of diet[84]. Tibia zinc and tibia ^{65}Zn were found[172] to be correlated with whole-body ^{65}Zn retention in rats fed chicken or soy-based diets containing 9 mg Zn/kg.

(g) Effect of testing conditions on absorption measurements

Testing conditions both before and after a meal can affect absorption measurements. Zinc absorption was lower in unfasted animals than in fasted ones, and the length of the fast was also important[173,174]. Absorption of Zn was lower in animals whose diet was reintroduced 2 h after the test meal than in animals refed 20 h later[173]. The Zn-content and general composition of the diet before the test meal can affect Zn absorption. Dietary Zn after a test meal affected Zn absorption by rats even when the meal was followed by a 7 h fast[173]. In humans, the volume of food in the meal, the volume of accompanying beverages, caloric content, whether food is solid or homogenized, and smoking, can affect gastric emptying time, and digestive secretions[175–178], and very probably affect intestinal transit time and mineral absorption.

As indicated elsewhere in this review, both the level of zinc in the diet and the dose of zinc in a meal can affect percentage zinc absorption. A dietary Zn–Zn dose interaction can affect the relative bioavailability of zinc from foods. When rats were fed basal diets containing 12 or 35 mg Zn/kg and 0.25 or 1.5 μmol Zn from zinc chloride, beef, chicken, peanut butter, milk, navy beans, oysters, and soybean flour, there were significant effects on zinc absorption of dietary Zn, Zn dose, Zn source, and a source–dose interaction[179]. Under certain conditions, zinc from chicken, beef, and zinc chloride was equally well absorbed, while under other conditions, zinc from chicken and peanut butter was more available than zinc from beef or zinc chloride. Likewise, zinc from navy beans was similar to, or significantly less available than, zinc chloride, depending on the usual dietary Zn and the Zn dose. Adaptation to other dietary components before the meal may also affect the outcome of absorption measurements. Rats adapted to a chicken meat diet absorbed more Zn from a soy test meal than rats adapted to a soy bean diet[172]. The zinc content of the diet fed after a test dose can also affect zinc absorption from that dose. Rats gavaged with carrier-free ^{65}Zn and subsequently fed a diet containing 11.5 mg Zn/kg absorbed more zinc than rats fed a diet containing 85 mg Zn/kg after the dose, when both groups were fed 85 mg Zn/kg before the test dose[180].

(h) Use of extrinsic labels

When isotopic tracers are used to measure zinc absorption from specific foods one must consider the validity of using an extrinsic tracer instead of an intrinsic tracer. An extrinsic tracer is an isotope which is added directly to the food at the time of meal preparation or feeding. An intrinsic tracer is one which is incorporated into a plant or animal during its normal growth before harvest or slaughter. The production of intrinsically labelled foods, especially with radioactive isotopes, is obviously cumbersome, and usually requires special facilities for the labelling process. However, extrinsic tracers, though convenient, must be proven to give the same results as intrinsic tracers. In rats, zinc absorption from intrinsic and extrinsic labels was comparable from rye grass[181], rat liver[182], corn[182], whole egg[183], chicken[172], soybean hulls[183], soybean flour[172,183,184] and neutralized soy concentrate[184]. Using an *in vitro* procedure, Sandström *et al.* concluded that extrinsic and intrinsic zinc were equally available from human milk[185]. Absorption of intrinsic zinc by rats was significantly lower than absorption of extrinsic zinc from acid-precipitated soy concentrate[184]. In humans, absorption of intrinsic zinc in chicken meat was significantly higher than absorption of extrinsic zinc added to chicken, although absorption of intrinsic and extrinsic zinc were significantly correlated[186]. However, other investigators found no difference between absorption of intrinsic and extrinsic zinc from turkey meat[187]. Absorption of intrinsic and extrinsic zinc from beef did not differ[188]. Solomons and Jacob used a plasma Zn tolerance procedure to compare the effects of different forms of iron on Zn absorption[166]. They found that non-haem iron inhibited the plasma Zn increase when Zn was given as zinc sulphate, but not when Zn was fed in the form of oysters. This raises the possibility that intrinsic and extrinsic zinc may not mix completely in the intestine, and can be affected to different degrees by substances which might enhance or inhibit Zn absorption.

3. Effects of foods and food components on zinc absorption

(a) Minerals

Other minerals in animal and human diets have been shown to interact with Zn and to affect its availability from the diet. Calcium has been shown to interfere with Zn absorption and retention by rats. Some investigators have observed a calcium effect only when diets were high in phytic acid or inorganic phosphorus[87,142], while others have reported an effect on calcium alone in reduction of zinc absorption[189]. Studies with humans have not shown an effect of calcium alone on zinc absorption[145]. Zinc absorption was reduced when milk was added to soy protein meal[190], but increased when milk was added to a meal with bread[170]. Both milk and cheese inhibited the rise in plasma zinc when pharmacological doses of zinc were fed to humans[164].

Zinc absorption is inhibited in humans by large excesses of inorganic iron over zinc[166] when salts of iron and zinc are given. Zinc absorption from food was not affected by large amounts of iron[191–193]. Haem iron did not affect the plasma appearance of pharmacological doses of zinc[166]. Inorganic iron affected plasma zinc increases after doses of zinc sulphate, but not zinc as oysters[166].

Copper can interfere with zinc absorption[194], but because diets usually contain much more zinc than copper, this effect is not usually considered important. A dose of 5 mg Cu did not interfere with absorption of 0.5 mg Zn as $ZnCl_2$ by humans[193].

(b) Vitamins

Folic acid supplements of 400 μg/d were shown[195] to increase faecal Zn excretion and decrease urinary Zn in men fed 3.5 mg Zn/d. However, in another study with men fed 8.5 mg Zn/d there was no difference in the absorption of Zn by men fed 200 or 400 μg folic acid/d, and an increase in Zn absorption when 800 μg/d of folic acid was given. Although Zn absorption increased at the high level of folic acid supplementation there was no change in Zn balance, suggesting that the increase in absorption was accompanied by a corresponding increase in endogenous fecal Zn excretion (PE Johnson and DB Milne, unpublished observations).

When pyridoxine HCl at concentrations of 2, 4, 10 and 40 mg/kg was added to rat diets, Zn absorption increased with increasing levels of dietary pyridoxine, and Zn turnover decreased[196].

Ascorbic acid had no effect on Zn absorption by human subjects[197] and had no effect on the rise in plasma zinc after a 25 mg dose of zinc[168].

(c) Proteins

The amount of protein in diets or meals affects the absorption and retention of zinc. Zinc retention by rats was improved when diets were high in total protein, and decreased when rats were fed low protein diets[198,199]. In humans, Sandström found that absorption of zinc was positively correlated with the protein content of meals[170].

The effect of protein sources on Zn absorption has been extensively studied, but it has not always been clear if the observed effects were caused by differences in the proteins themselves, or in other food components such as phytic acid. The requirement for dietary Zn in the rat is 12 mg/kg when casein is used as the protein source, but 18 mg/kg when soy flour is used[17]. Conflicting data on the effects of soy protein on zinc availability may reflect differences in zinc levels in the chronic diet, prior adaptation to soy protein-containing diets, the phytate: zinc molar ratio, the type of soy product fed[172,183,184,200–202]. (Phytic acid is present to some degree even in the processed soy products.) In humans, zinc absorption from soy-based infant formula was less than from human or cow's milk[62,63], but addition of soy to a milk formula did not depress zinc absorption[62]. Only 30% of zinc was absorbed from a soy bean sausage meal, but 41% was absorbed from a meal of beef sausage[197]. Zinc absorption by humans fed a formula diet containing chicken was 57–72%, at Zn intakes of 10.1 or 6.7 mg Zn/d[186], and replacement of half the chicken by soy did not affect Zn absorption. In contrast, replacement of meat or protein in bread by soy in bread by soy products depressed Zn absorption from test meals[203].

Zinc is better absorbed from human milk than from cow's milk or cow's milk-based infant formula[61–63]. This difference has been attributed to low molecular weight zinc binding substances in human milk which are absent or at low levels in cow's milk[30,42–44]. Significantly more ^{65}Zn was retained by rats fed a whey-based diet (36.5%) than by rats fed a casein-based diet (31.6%); femur zinc and ^{65}Zn were also higher in rats fed the whey diet[204]. In humans, zinc absorption from a 'humanized' cow's milk infant formula (whey/casein 60/40) was significantly higher than from a conventional (whey/casein 20/80) formula (32% vs. 21%); however, absorption from a 100% casein formula (41%) was higher than from a 100% whey formula (26.5%)[62].

In rats, zinc was better absorbed from chicken than from beef[179], but in humans, zinc absorption from chicken and beef was similar when zinc was added to chicken to equalize the amount of zinc in the chicken and beef meals[190]. Human zinc absorption from beef, chicken, and turkey meals containing 1.0–5.0 mg Zn ranged from 20 to 41%[190].

119

Zinc availability is generally, but not always, better from foods of animal origin than from foods of plant origin. O'Dell first compared plant and animal foods using growth-response as a criterion, and found zinc from egg yolk, fish meal, oysters, and non-fat dry milk to be more available than zinc from corn, rice, wheat, corn germ, sesame meal, or soybean meal[205]. Zinc absorption by rats from peanut butter was equal to or significantly higher than that from zinc sulphate, depending on conditions of dose and dietary Zn[179]. Zinc absorption by rats from egg or chicken was better than from soy protein[179].

(d) Plant foods

Breads and cereals, as well as legumes, have been studied extensively because they are dietary staples. Human zinc deficiency was first recognized in the Middle East where unleavened whole-wheat breads comprise much of the diet[206]. These breads are rich in both fibre and phytate.

There is substantial evidence that phytate added to diets inhibits the absorption of zinc by rats[207,208]. Dephytinization of bran reduces its inhibitory effects on zinc absorption[209]. Reduction of phytates content of bread by leavening also improves zinc availability for absorption[210]. Stable isotope studies in humans showed a 50% reduction in Zn absorption when 3 g of sodium phytate/d were added to the diet[211].

Fibre in the form of bran has been found to reduce zinc absorption and retention[212,213] or to have no effect[214,215]. The particle size of the bran was suggested to be a factor in these conflicting results[216], but particle size does not always have an effect[215]. In humans, zinc absorption from wholemeal bread was less than half (17%) of that from white bread (38%), but the zinc content of the wholemeal bread was three times that of the white bread, so that the total zinc absorbed was greater from the wholemeal bread[170]. Pecoud et al.[164] found that brown bread inhibited the rise in plasma zinc to a greater extent than did white bread. Addition of cellulose to a formula diet did not affect zinc absorption in humans as measured with stable isotopes[211].

Oxalic acid, found in leafy green vegetables, does not affect absorption of zinc by rats[217].

(e) Beverages

Red wine enhanced zinc balance in humans[218]. This effect was caused by the congeners rather than the ethanol, as dealcoholized wine had the same effect. Wine, whiskey, or beer served with a turkey meal did not affect zinc absorption[187]. Ethanol-feeding studies in rats, which allow consumption at high levels of alcohol for prolonged periods, have shown a reduction of zinc absorption and increased zinc excretion in ethanol-fed rats[219,220].

Milk served with turkey caused a small but non-significant reduction in zinc absorption[187]. Milk added to a meal of wholemeal bread and egg resulted in a small increase in zinc absorption[170]. Zinc is better absorbed from human milk than from cow's milk[61–63].

Orange juice depressed zinc absorption from a meal of turkey[187]. Coffee inhibited plasma zinc uptake after a pharmacological dose of zinc[211], but tea taken with a meal of turkey did not affect zinc absorption by humans[187].

SUMMARY

Although we know more about the absorption and excretion of zinc than other other trace minerals, such as copper, knowledge of the mechanisms involved is still fragmentary. From a practical standpoint much remains to be learned about the bioavailability of zinc from foods consumed in ordinary diets. Much of the existing data is conflicting or incomplete. Rapid advances in methodologies with both stable and radioactive isotopes in the past decade are beginning to give us information about zinc absorption by healthy people.

References

1. Van Campen, DR and Mitchell, EA (1965). Absorption of Cu^{64}, Zn^{65}, Mo^{99}, and Fe^{59} from ligated segments of the rat gastrointestinal tract. *J Nutr*, **86**, 120–124

2. Methfessel, AH and Spencer, H (1973). Zinc metabolism in the rat, I. Intestinal absorption of zinc. *J Appl Physiol*, **34**, 58–62

3. Davies, NT (1980). Studies on the absorption of zinc by rat intestine. *Br J Nutr*, **43**, 189–203

4. Hampton, DL, Miller, WJ, Neathery, MW *et al.* (1976). Intestinal sites of zinc absorption as determined by direct ^{64}Zn dosing of intact rats. *Nutr Rept Int*, **14**, 691–697

5. Ghishan, FK and Sobo, G (1983). Intestinal maturation: *in vivo* zinc transport. *Paediatr Res*, **17**, 148–151

6. Sahagian, BM, Harding-Barlow, I and Perry, HM (1966). Uptakes of zinc, manganese, cadmium and mercury by intact strips of rat intestine. *J Nutr*, **90**, 259–267

7. Atonson, DL, Barak, AJ and Vanderhoof, JA (1979). Determination of the site of zinc absorption in rat small intestine. *J Nutr*, **109**, 142–147

8. Matseshe, JW, Phillips, SF, Malagelada, JR and McCall, JT (1980). Recovery of dietary iron and zinc from the proximal intestine of healthy man: studies of different meals and supplements. *Am J Clin Nutr*, **33**, 1946–1953

9. Sandström, B, Cederblad, A, Kivistö *et al.* (1986). Retention of zinc and calcium from the human colon. *Am J Clin Nutr*, **44**, 501–504

10. Meneely, R and Ghishan, FK (1982). *In vivo* intestinal zinc transport in rats: normal and growth retarded. *J Pediatr Gastroenterol Nutr*, **1**, 119–124

11. Kowarski, S, Blais-Stanek, CS and Schacter, D (1974). Active transport of zinc and identification of zinc-binding protein in rat jejunal mucosa. *Am J Physiol*, **226**, 401–407

12. Marcus, CS and Lengemann, FW (1962). Use of radioyttrium to study food movement in the small intestine of the rat. *J Nutr*, **76**, 179–182

13. Steel, L and Cousins, RJ (1985). Kinetics of zinc absorption by luminally and vascularly perfused rat intestine. *Am J Physiol*, **248**, G46–G53

14. Menard, MP and Cousins, RJ (1983). Zinc transport by brush border membrane vesicles from rat intestine. *J Nutr*, **113**, 1434–1442

15. Kirchgessner, M and Weigand, E (1983). Zinc absorption and excretion in relation to nutrition. In Siegel, H (ed.), *Zinc and its Role in Biology and Nutrition. Metal ions in biological systems*, Vol.15, pp. 319–362 (New York: Marcel Dekker)

16. Leucke, RW, Olman, ME and Baltzer, BV (1968). Zinc deficiency in the rat. *J Nutr*, **94**, 344–350

17. Forbes, RM and Yohe, M (1960). Zinc requirement and balance studies with the rat. *J Nutr*, **70**, 53–57

18. Hamilton, DL, Bellamy, JEC, Valberg, JD and Valberg, LS (1978). Zinc, cadmium, and iron interactions during intestinal absorption in iron-deficient mice. *Can J Physiol Pharmacol*, **56**, 384–389

19. Flanagan, PR, Haist, J and Valberg, LS (1983). Zinc absorption, intraluminal zinc and intestinal metallothionein levels in zinc-replete rodents. *J Nutr*, **113**, 962–972

20. Steinhardt, HJ and Adibi, SA (1984). Interaction between transport of zinc and other solutes in human intestine. *Am J Physiol*, **247**, G176–G182

21. Menard, MP, Oestreicher, P and Cousins, RJ (1983). Zinc transport by isolated, vascularly perfused rat intestine and brush border vesicles. In Inglett, GC (ed.), *Nutritional Bioavailability of Zinc*. ACS Symposium Series, pp. 233–246 (Washington DC: American Chemical Society)

22. Wapnir, RA and Stiel, L (1986). Zinc intestinal absorption in rats: Specificity of amino acids as ligands. *J Nutr*, **116**, 2171–2179

23. Hahn, C and Evans, GW (1973). Identification of a low molecular weight ^{65}Zn complex in rat intestine. *Proc Soc Exp Biol Med*, **144**, 793–795

24. Evans, GW, Grace, CI and Votava, HJ (1975). A proposed mechanism for zinc absorption in the rat. *Am J Physiol*, **228**, 501–505

25. Evans, GW and Hahn, CJ (1975). Copper and zinc-binding components in rat intestine. In Friedman, M (ed.), *Protein Interactions*, pp. 285–297 (New York: Plenum)

26. Richards, MP and Cousins, RJ (1975). Influence of parenteral zinc and actinomycin D on tissue zinc uptake and the synthesis of a zinc-binding protein. *Bioinorg Chem*, **4**, 215–224

27. Hahn, CJ, Severson, ML and Evans, GW (1976). Structure of a zinc ligand isolated from duodenum. *Fed Proc*, **35**, 863

28. Evans, GW and Johnson, PE (1978). Ligands involved in the intestinal absorption of copper and zinc. In Kirchgessner, M (ed.), *Trace Element Metabolism in Man and Animals*, Vol.III, pp. 98–105 (Werhenstephan: Arbeitskreis für Tierernährungsforschung)

29. Song, MK and Adham, NF (1978). Role of prostaglandin E2 in zinc absorption in the rat. *Am J Physiol*, **234**, E99–E105

30. Evans, GW, Johnson, PE and Johnson, EC (1979). Purification and characterization of a zinc-binding ligand in rat intestine. *J Nutr*, **109**, xxxiii

31. Evans, GW (1983). Picolinic acid and zinc absorption. In Sarkar, B (ed.), *Biological Aspects of Metals and Metal-Related Diseases*, pp. 81–88 (New York: Raven Press)

32. Cousins, RJ, Smith, KT, Failla, ML and Markowitz, LA (1978). Origin of low molecular weight zinc-binding complexes from ligands in rat intestine. *Life Sci*, **23**, 1819–1826

33. Song, MK and Adham, NF (1979). Evidence for an important role of prostaglandins E2 and F2 in the regulation of zinc transport in the rat. *J Nutr*, **109**, 2152–2159

34. Sillen, LG and Martell, AE (1964). *Stability Constants of Metal–Ion Complexes*. Special Publication No.17 (London: Chemical Society)

35. Seal, CJ and Heaton, FW (1983). Chemical factors affecting the intestinal absorption of zinc *in vitro* and *in vivo*. *Br J Nutr*, **50**, 317–324

36. Seal, CJ and Heaton, FW (1985). Effect of dietary picolinic acid on the metabolism of exogenous and endogenous zinc in the rat. *J Nutr*, **115**, 986–993

37. Wapnir, RA, Khani, DE, Bayne, MA and Lifshitz, F (1983). Absorption of zinc by the rat ileum: effects of histidine and other low-molecular weight ligands. *J Nutr*, 113, 1346–1354
38. Oestreicher, P and Cousins, RJ (1982). Influence of intraluminal constituents on zinc absorption by isolated, vascularly perfused rat intestine. *J Nutr*, 112, 1978–1982
39. Jackson, MJ, Jones, DA and Edwards, RHT (1981). Zinc absorption in the rat. *Br J Nutr*, 46, 15–27
40. Evans, GW and Johnson, EC (1980). Zinc absorption in rats fed a low-protein diet and a low-protein diet supplemented with tryptophan or picolinic acid. *J Nutr*, 110, 1076–1080
41. Evans, GW (1980). Normal and abnormal zinc absorption in man and animals: the tryptophan connection. *Nutr Rev*, 38, 137–141
42. Evans, GW and Johnson, PE (1976). Zinc-binding factor in acrodermatitis enteropathica. *Lancet*, 2, 1310
43. Eckhert, CD, Sloan, MV, Duncan, JR and Hurley, LS (1976). Zinc binding: A difference between human and bovine milk. *Science*, 195, 789–790
44. Hurley, LS, Duncan, JR, Sloan, MV and Eckhert, CD (1977). Zinc-binding ligands in milk and intestine: A role in neonatal nutrition. *Proc Natl Acad Sci USA*, 74, 3574–3549
45. Evans, GW and Johnson, PE (1980). Characterization and quantitation of a zinc-binding ligand in human milk. *Pediatr Res*, 14, 876–880
46. Hurley, LS, Lonnerdal, B and Stanislowski, AG (1979). Zinc citrate, human milk, and acrodermatitis enteropathica. *Lancet*, 1, 677–678
47. Lonnderdal, B, Stanislowski, AG and Hurley, LS (1980). Isolation of a low molecular weight zinc binding ligand from human milk. *J Inorg Biochem*, 12, 71–78
48. Martin, MT, Licklider, KF, Brushmiller, JG and Jacobs, FA (1981). Detection of low molecular weight copper(II) and zinc(II) ligands in ultrafiltered milk – the citrate connection. *J Inorg Biochem*, 15, 55–65
49. Neldner, KH, Hambidge, KM and Walravens, PA (1978). Acrodermatitis enteropathica. *Intl J Dermatol*, 17, 380–385
50. Atherton, DJ, Muller, DPR, Aggett, PJ and Harries, JT (1979). A defect in zinc uptake by jejunal biopsies in acrodermatitis enteropathica. *Clin Sci*, 56, 505–507
51. Simell, O, Rahola, T, Suomela, M et al. (1978). Zinc absorption and losses in acrodermatitis enteropathica (AE) using total body counting for ^{65}Zn detection. *Acta Paediatr Belg*, 31, 257
52. Weismann, K, Hoe, S, Knudsen, L and Sorenson, SS (1979). ^{65}Zinc absorption in patients suffering from acrodermatitis enteropathica and in normal adults assessed by whole-body counting technique. *Br J Dermatol*, 101, 573–579
53. Duncan, JR and Hurley, LS (1978). Intestinal absorption of zinc: a role for a zinc-binding ligand in milk. *Am J Physiol*, 235, E556–E559
54. Krieger, I, Cash, R and Evans, GW (1984). Picolinic acid in acrodermatitis enteropathica: evidence for a disorder of tryptophan metabolism. *J Pediatr Gastoenterol Nutr*, 3, 62–68
55. Piletz, JE and Ganschow, GE (1979). Is acrodermatitis enteropathica related to the absence of zinc binding ligand in human milk? *Am J Clin Nutr*, 32, 275–281
56. Cousins, RJ and Smith, KT (1980). Zinc-binding properties of bovine and human milk *in vitro*: influence of changes in zinc content. *Am J Clin Nutr*, 33, 1083–1087
57. Rebello, T, Lonnerdal, B and Hurley, LS (1982). Picolinic acid in milk, pancreatic juice, and intestine: inadequate for role in zinc absorption. *Am J Clin Nutr*, 35, 1–5
58. Holt, C (1981). Zinc binding ligands in milk: Both arguments err seriously. *J Nutr*, 111, 2240–2242
59. Hurley, LS and Lonnerdal, B (1982). Zinc binding in human milk: citrate versus picolinate. *Nutr Rev*, 40, 65–71

60.   Evans, GW (1980). Normal and abnormal zinc absorption in man and animals: the tryptophan connection. *Nutr Rev*, **38**, 137–141

61.   Johnson, PE and Evans, GW (1978). Relative zinc availability in human breast milk, infant formulas, and cow's milk. *Am J Clin Nutr*, **31**, 416–421

62.   Sandstrom, B, Cederblad, A and Lonnerdal, B (1983). Zinc absorption from human milk, cow's milk, and infant formulas. *Am J Dis Child*, **137**, 726–729

63.   Casey, CE, Walravens, PA and Hambidge, KM (1981). Availability of zinc: loading tests with human milk, cow's milk, and infant formulas. *Pediatrics*, **68**, 394–396

64.   Cousins, RJ (1979). Regulation of zinc absorption: role of intracellular ligands. *Am J Clin Nutr*, **32**, 339–335

65.   Solomons, NW and Cousins, RJ (1984). Zinc. In Solomons, NW and Rosenberg, IH (eds), *Absorption and Malabsorption of Mineral Nutrients*, pp. 125–197 (New York: Liss)

66.   Cousins, RJ (1979). Regulatory aspects of zinc metabolism in liver and intestine. *Nutr Rev*, **37**, 97–103

67.   Cousins, RJ (1985). Absorption, transport, and hepatic metabolism of copper and zinc: special reference to metallothionein and ceruloplasmin. *Physiol Rev*, **65**, 238–308

68.   Starcher, BC (1969). Studies on the mechanism of copper absorption in the chick. *J Nutr*, **97**, 321–326

69.   Evans, GW, Majors, PF and Cornatzer, WE (1970). Mechanism for cadmium and zinc antagonism of copper metabolism. *Biochem Biophys Res Commun*, **40**, 1142–1148

70.   Van Campen, DR and Kowalski, TJ (1971). Studies on zinc absorption: [65]Zn binding by homogenates of rat intestinal mucosa. *Proc Soc Exp Biol Med*, **136**, 294–297

71.   Richards, MP and Cousins, RJ (1977). Isolation of an intestinal metallothionein induced by parenteral zinc. *Biochem Biophys Res Commun*, **75**, 286–294

72.   Richards, MP and Cousins, RJ (1976). Zinc-binding protein: relationship to short term changes in zinc metabolism. *Proc Soc Exp Biol Med*, **153**, 52–56

73.   Richards, MP and Cousins, RJ (1976). Metallothionein and its relationship to the metabolism of dietary zinc in rats. *J Nutr*, **106**, 1591–1599

74.   Richards, MP and Cousins, RJ (1975). Influence of parenteral zinc and actinomycin D on tissue zinc uptake and the synthesis of a zinc-binding protein. *Bioinorg Chem*, **4**, 215–224

75.   Menard, MP, McCormich, CC and Cousins, RJ (1981). Regulation of intestinal metallothionein biosynthesis in rats by dietary zinc. *J Nutr*, **111**, 1353–1361

76.   Richards, MP and Cousins, RJ (1975). Mammalian zinc homeostasis: requirements for RNA and metallothionein synthesis. *Biochem Biophys Res Commun*, **64**, 1215–1223

77.   Hall, AC, Young, BW and Bremner, I (1979). Intestinal metallothionein and the mutual antagonism between copper and zinc in the rat. *J Inorg Biochem*, **11**, 57–66

78.   Olafson, RW (1983). Intestinal metallothionein: effect of parenteral and enteral zinc exposure on tissue levels of mice on controlled diets. *J Nutr*, **113**, 268–275

79.   Song, MK, Adham, NF and Ament, ME (1986). Relative zinc-binding activities of ligands in the cytosol of rat small intestine. *Comp Biochem Physiol*, **85C**, 283–289

80.   Coppen, DE and Davies, NT (1987). Studies on the effects of dietary zinc dose on [65]Zinc absorption *in vivo* and the effects of Zn status on [65]Zn absorption and body loss in young rats. *Br J Nutr*, **57**, 35–44

81.   Hunt, JR, Johnson, PE and Swan, PB (1987). The influence of usual zinc intake and zinc in a meal on [65]Zn retention and turnover in the rat. *J Nutr* **117**, 1427–1433

82.   Seal, CJ and Heaton, FW (1987). Zinc transfer among proteins in rat duodenum mucosa. *Ann Nutr Metab*, **31**, 55–60

83.   Pallauf, J and Kirchgessner, M (1972). Zinkehalte in Knochen und Ganzkorper

wachsender ratten bei unterschiedlicher Zinkversorgung. *Z Tierphysiol Tiernährg u Futtermittelkde*, **30**, 193–202

84. Deeming, SB and Weber, CW (1977). Evaluation of hair analysis for determination of zinc status using rats. *Am J Clinc Nutr*, **30**, 2047–2052

85. Cotzias, GC, Borg, DC and Selleck, B (1962). Specificity of zinc pathway through the body: turnover of Zn^{65} in the mouse. *Am J Physiol*, **202**, 359–363

86. Furchner, JE and Richmond, CR (1962). Effect of dietary zinc on the absorption of orally administered ^{64}Zn. *Health Phys*, **8**, 35–40

87. Heth, DA, Becker, WM and Hoekstra, WG (1966). Effect of calcium, phosphorus, and zinc on zinc-65 absorption and turnover in rats fed semipurified diets. *J Nutr*, **88**, 331–337

88. Rubini, ME, Montalvo, G, Lockhart, CP and Johnson, CR (1961). Metabolism of zinc-65. *Am J Physiol*, **200**, 1345–1348

89. Weigand, E and Kirchgessner, M (1977). Model study on the factorial derivation of the requirement of trace elements. Zinc requirement of the growing rat. *Z Tierphysiol Tiernährg u Futtermittelkde*, **39**, 84–95

90. Weigand, E and Kirchgessner, M (1978). Homeostatic adjustments in zinc digestion to widely varying dietary zinc intake. *Nutr Metab*, **22**, 101–112

91. Weigand, E and Kirchgessner, M (1980). Total true efficiency of zinc utilization: determination and homeostatic dependence upon the zinc supply status in young rats. *J Nutr*, **110**, 469–480

92. Evans, GW, Johnson, EC and Johnson, PE (1979). Zinc absorption in the rat determined by radioisotope dilution. *J Nutr*, **109**, 1258–1264

93. Miller, WJ, Blackmon, DM, Gentry, RP *et al.* (1967). Absorption, excretion, and retention of orally administered zinc-65 in various tissues of zinc-deficient and normal goats and calves. *J Nutr*, **92**, 71–78

94. Miller, WJ, Martin, YG, Gentry, RP and Blackmon, DM (1968). ^{65}Zn and stable zinc absorption, excretion and tissue concentrations as affected by type of diet and level of zinc in normal calves. *J Nutr*, **94**, 391–401

95. Istfan, NW, Janghorbani, M and Young, VR (1983). Absorption of stable ^{70}Zn in healthy young men in relation to zinc intake. *Am J Clin Nutr*, **38**, 187–194

96. Wada, L, Turnlund, JR and King, JC (1985). Zinc utilization in young men fed adequate and low zinc intakes. *J Nutr*, **115**, 1345–1354

97. Miller, WJ, Blackmon, DM, Powell, GW *et al.* (1966). Effects of zinc deficiency *per se* and of dietary zinc level on urinary and endogenous fecal excretion of ^{65}Zn from a single intravenous dose by ruminants. *J Nutr*, **90**, 335–341

98. Aamodt, RL, Rumble, WF, Babcock, AK *et al.* (1982). Effect of oral zinc loading on zinc metabolism in humans. I. Experimental studies. *Metabolism*, **31**, 326–334

99. Patron, KB, Flanagan, PR, Stinson, EA *et al.* (1982). Technique for determination of human zinc absorption from measurement of radioactivity in a fecal sample of the body. *Gastroenterology*, **83**, 1264–1270

100. Weigand, E and Kirchgessner, M (1976). Radioisotope dilution technique for determination of zinc absorption *in vivo*. *Nutr Metab*, **20**, 307–313

101. Johnson, PE, Hunt, JR and Ralston, NVC (1987). The effect of body zinc stores and current diet on true absorption, endogenous excretion, and zinc balance in rats. *Fed Proc*, **46**, 600

102. Wastney, ME, Aamodt, RL, Rumble, WF and Henkin, RE (1986). Kinetic analysis of zinc metabolism and its regulation in normal humans. *Am J Physiol*, **251**, R398–R408

103. Johnson, PE and Evans, GW (1980). Source of maternal milk zinc for absorption by suckling rats. *Proc Soc Exp Biol Med*, **163**, 372–375

104. Neathery, MW, Miller, WP, Blackmon, DM *et al.* (1973). Absorption and tissue zinc content in lactating dairy cows as affected by low dietary zinc. *J Anim Sci*, **37**, 848–852

105. Hill, GM, Miller, ER and Ku, PK (1985). Effect of dietary zinc levels on mineral concentration in milk. *J Anim Sci*, **57**, 123–129

106. Mutch, PB and Hurley, LS (1974). Effect of zinc deficiency during lactation on postnatal growth and development of rats. *J Nutr*, **104**, 828–842

107. Miller, WJ, Clifton, CM, Fowler, PR and Perkins, HF (1966). Influence of high levels of dietary zinc on zinc in milk, performance, and biochemistry of lactating cows. *J Dairy Sci*, **48**, 450–453

108. Vaughan, LA, Weber, CW and Kemberling, SR (1979). Longitudinal changes in the mineral content of human milk. *Am J Clin Nutr*, **32**, 2301–2306

109. Vuori, E, Makinen, SM, Kara, R and Kuitunen, P (1980). The effects of the dietary intakes of copper, iron, manganese, and zinc on the trace element content of human milk. *Am J Clin Nutr*, **33**, 227–231

110. Feely, RM, Eitenmiller, RR, Jones, JB, Jr and Barnhart, H (1983). Copper, iron, and zinc contents of human milk at early stages of lactation. *Am J Clin Nutr*, **37**, 443–448

111. Moser, PB and Reynolds, RD (1983). Dietary zinc intake and zinc concentrations of plasma, erythrocytes, and breast milk in antepartum and postpartum lactating and nonlactating women: a longitudinal study. *Am J Clin Nutr*, **38**, 101–108

112. Moore, MEC, Moran, JR and Greene, HL (1984). Zinc supplementation in lactating women: evidence for mammary control of zinc secretion. *J Pediatr*, **105**, 600–602

113. Milne, DB, Canfield, WK, Mahalko, JR and Sandstead, HH (1983). Effect of dietary zinc on whole body surface loss of zinc impact on estimation of zinc retention by balance method. *Am J Clin Nutr*, **38**, 181–186

114. Prasad, AS, Schubert, AR, Sandstead, HH *et al.* (1963). Zinc, iron, and nitrogen content of sweat in normal and deficient subjects. *J Lab Clin Med*, **62**, 84–89

115. Ott, EA, Smith, WH, Stob, M and Beeson, WM (1964). Zinc deficiency syndrome in the young lamb. *J Nutr*, **82**, 41–50

116. Reinhold, JG, Kfoury, GA and Thomas, TA (1967). Zinc, copper and iron concentrations in hair and other tissues: effects of low zinc and low protein intakes in rats. *J Nutr*, **92**, 173–182

117. Klevay, LM (1970). Hair as a biopsy material. I. Assessment of zinc nutriture. *Am J Clin Nutr*, **23**, 284–289

118. McKenzie, J (1979). Content of zinc in serum, urine, hair, and toenails of New Zealand adults. *Am J Clin Nutr*, **32**, 570–579

119. Umoren, J and Kies, C (1982). Menstrual blood losses of iron, zinc, copper and magnesium in adult female subjects. *Nutr Rept Int*, **26**, 717–726

120. Hess, FM, King, J and Margen, S (1976). The effect of a low zinc intake on zinc excretion in healthy young women. *Fed Proc*, **35**, 2494

121. Greger, JL and Buckley, S (1977). Menstrual loss of zinc, copper, magnesium and iron by adolescent girls. *Nutr Rept Int*, **16**, 639–647

122. Schroeder, HA, Nason, AP, Tipton, IH and Balussa JJ (1967). Essential trace elements in man: Zinc. Relation to environmental cadmium. *J Chron Dis*, **20**, 179–210

123. Marmar, JL, Katy, S, Praiss, DE and DeBenedictus, TJ (1975). Semen zinc levels in infertile and postvasectomy patients and patients with prostatitis. *Fertil Steril*, **26**, 1057–1063

124. Marmar, JL, Katz, S, Praiss, DE and DeBenedictus, TJ (1980). Values for zinc in whole semen, fractions of split ejaculate, and expressed prostatic fluid. *Urology*, **26**, 478–80

125. Baer, MT and King, JC (1984). Tissue zinc levels and zinc excretion during experimental zinc depletion in young men. *Am J Clin Nutr*, **39**, 556–570

126. Aamodt, RL and Rumble, WF (1983). Zinc absorption in humans. Effects of age, sex, and food. In Inglett, GE (ed.), *Nutritional Bioavailability of Zinc*, pp. 61–82. ACS Symposium Series No. 210. (Washington DC: American Chemical Society)

127. Turnlund, JR, Michel, MC, Keyes, WR *et al.* (1982). Use of enriched stable isotopes to determine zinc and iron absorption in young men. *Am J Clin Nutr*, **35**, 1033–1040

128. Wada, L, Turnlund, JR and King, JC (1985). Zinc utilization in young men fed adequate and low zinc intakes. *J Nutr*, 115, 1345–1354
129. Schwarz, FJ, Kirchgessner, M and Sherif, SY (1981). Zur intestinalen absorption von zinc während der Gravidität und Laktation. *Res Exp Med (Berl)*, 179, 35–42
130. Swanson, CA, Turnlund, JR and King, JC (1983). Effect of dietary zinc sources and pregnancy on zinc utilization in adult women fed controlled diets. *J Nutr*, 1113, 2557–2567
131. Dinsmore, W, Callender, ME, McMaster, D *et al.* (1985). Zinc absorption in alcoholics using zinc-65. *Digestion*, 32, 238–242
132. Sturniolo, GC, Molokhia, MM, Shields, R and Turnberg, LA (1980). Zinc absorption in Crohn's disease. *Gut*, 21, 387–391
133. Valberg, LS, Flanagan, PR, Kerstesz, A and Bondy, DC (1986). Zinc absorption in inflammatory bowel disease. *Dig Dis Sci*, 31, 724–731
134. Boosalis, M, Evans, G and McClain, C (1983). Impaired handling of orally administered zinc in pancreatic insufficiency. *Am J Clin Nutr*, 37, 268–271
135. Dinsmore, WW, Alderdice, JT, McMaster, D *et al.* (1985). Zinc absorption in anorexia nervosa. *Lancet*, 1, 1041–1042
136. Lombeck, I, Schnippering, HC, Ritzl, F *et al.* (1975). Absorption of zinc in acrodermatitis enteropathica. *Lancet*, 1, 855
137. Henken, RI and Aamodt, RL (1975). Zinc absorption in acrodermatitis in hypogeusia and hyposmia. *Lancet*, 1, 137
138. Flagstad, T (1976). Lethal trait A46 in cattle. Intestinal zinc absorption. *Nord Vet Med*, 28, 60–169
139. Flagstad, T (1981). Zinc absorption in cattle with a dietary picolinic acid supplement. *J Nutr*, 111, 1996–1999
140. Ghishan, FK and Greene, HL (1983). Intestinal transport of zinc in the diabetic rat. *Life Sci*, 32, 1735–1741
141. Walravens, PA (1979). Zinc metabolism and its implications in clinical medicine. *West J Med*, 130, 133–142
142. Heth, DA and Hoekstra, WG (1965). Zinc-65 absorption and turnover in rats. I. A procedure to determine zinc-65 absorption and the antagonistic effect of calcium in a practical diet. *J Nutr*, 85, 367–374
143. Arvidsson, B, Cederblad, Å, Björn-Rasmussen, E and Sandström, B (1978). A radionuclide technique for studies of zinc absorption in man. *Int J Nucl Med Biol*, 5, 109–113
144. Lykken, GI (1983). A whole body counting technique using ultralow doses of ^{59}Fe and [65]Zn in absorption and retention studies in humans. *Am J Clin Nutr*, 37, 652–662
145. Spencer, H, Vankinscott, V, Lewin, I and Samachson, J (1965). Zinc-65 metabolism during low and high calcium intake in man. *J Nutr*, 86, 169–177
146. Spencer, H, Rosoff, B and Feldstein, A (1965). Metabolism of zinc-65 in man. *Radiat Res*, 24, 432–445
147. Foster, DM, Aamodt, RL, Henken, RI and Berman, M (1979). Zinc metabolism in humans: a kinetic model. *Am J Physiol*, 237, R340–R349
148. Foster, DM, Wastney, ME and Henken, RI (1984). Zinc metabolism in humans: a kinetic model. *Math Biosci*, 72, 359–372
149. Aamodt, RL, Rumble, WF, Johnston, GS *et al.* (1979). Zinc metabolism in humans after oral and intravenous administration of Zn-69m. *Am J Clin Nutr*, 32, 559–569
150. Richmond, CR, Furchner, JE, Trafton, GA and Langham, WH (1962). Comparative metabolism of radionuclides in mammals. I. Uptake and retention of orally administered [65]Zn by four mammalian species. *Health Phys*, 8, 481–489
151. Payton, KB, Flanagan, PR, Stinson, EA *et al.* (1982). Technique for determination of human zinc absorption from measurement of radioactivity in a fecal sample of the body. *Gastroenterology*, 83, 1264–1270
152. Janghorbani, M, Ting, BTG and Young, VR (1980). Accurate analysis of stable iso-

tope ^{68}Zn, ^{70}Zn and ^{58}Fe in human feces with neutron activation analysis. *Clin Chem Acta*, **108**, 9–24

153. Janghorbani, M and Young, VR (1980). Use of stable isotopes to determine bioavailability of minerals in human diets using the method of fecal monitoring. *Am J Clin Nutr*, **33**, 2021–2030

154. Janghorbani, M, Young, VR, Gramlich, JW and Machlan, LA (1981). Comparative measurements of Zinc-70 enrichment in human plasma samples with neutron activation and mass spectrometry. *Clin Chem Acta*, **114**, 163–171

155. Johnson, PE (1982). A mass spectrometric method for use of stable isotopes as tracers in studies of iron, zinc, and copper absorption in human subjects. *J Nutr*, **112**, 1414–1424

156. Hachey, DL, Blais, JC and Klein, PD (1980). High precision isotopic ratio analysis of volatile metal chelates. *Anal Chem*, **52**, 1131–1135

157. Pierce, P, Hambidge, M, Fennessey, P *et al.* (1987). Evaluation of zinc (Zn) absorption in the preterm infant using a stable isotope technique. *Fed Proc*, **46**, 748

158. Turnlund, JR, Michel, MC *et al.* (1982). Use of enriched stable isotopes to determine zinc and iron absorption in elderly men. *Am J Clin Nutr*, **35**, 1033–1040

159. Klitenich, MA, Frederichson, CJ and Manton, WI (1983). Acid-vapor decomposition for determination of zinc in brain tissue by isotope dilution mass spectrometry. *Anal Chem*, **55**, 921–923

160. Gotz, A and Heumann, KG (1987). Schwermetall-spurenbestimmung mit einem Kompakten Thermionen-Quadrupol-Massenspektrometer Teil 2. Analyse von Lebensmittelproben. *Fresenius Z Anal Chem*, **326**, 118–122

161. Lo, GS, Steinke, FH, Ting, BTG *et al.* (1981). Comparative measurement of zinc absorption in rats with stable isotope ^{70}Zn and radioisotope ^{65}Zn. *J Nutr*, **111**, 2236–2239

162. Janghorbani, M, Ting, BTG, Istfan, NW and Young, VR (1981). Measurement of ^{68}Zn and ^{70}Zn in human blood in reference to the study of zinc metabolism. *Am J Clin Nutr*, **34**, 581–591

163. Jackson, MJ, Jones, DA, Edwards, RHT *et al.* (1984). Zinc homeostasis in man: studies using a new stable isotope-dilution technique. *Br J Nutr*, **51**, 199–208

164. Pecóud, A, Donzel, P and Schelling, JL (1975). Effect of foodstuffs on the absorption of zinc sulfate. *Clin Pharm Therap*, **12**, 469–474

165. Sullivan, JF, Jetton, MM and Burch, RE (1979). A zinc tolerance test. *J Lab Clin Med*, **93**, 485–492

166. Solomons, NW and Jacobs, RA (1981). Studies on the bioavailability of zinc in humans: effects of heme and nonheme iron on the absorption of zinc. *Am J Clin Nutr*, **34**, 475–482

167. Solomons, NW, Jacob, RA, Pineda, O and Viteri, F (1979). Studies on the bioavailability of zinc in man. II. Absorption of zinc from organic and inorganic sources. *J Lab Clin Med*, **94**, 335–343

168. Solomons, NW, Jacob, RA, Pineda, O and Viteri, FE (1979). Studies on the bioavailability of zinc in man. III. Effects of ascorbic acid on zinc absorption. *Am J Clin Nutr*, **32**, 2495–2499

169. Solomons, NW, Pineda, O, Viteri, F and Sandstead, HH (1983). Studies on the bioavailability of zinc in humans: mechanisms of intestinal interaction of honheme iron and zinc. *J Nutr*, **113**, 337–349

170. Sandström, B, Arvidsson, B, Cederblad, Å and Björn-Rasmussen, E (1980). Zinc absorption from composite meals. I. The significance of wheat extraction rate, zinc, calcium, and protein content in meals based on bread. *Am J Clin Nutr*, **33**, 739–745

171. Valberg, LS, Flanagan, PR, Brennan, J and Chamberlain, MJ (1985). Does the oral zinc tolerance test measure zinc absorption? *J Clin Nutr*, **41**, 37–42

172. Stuart, SM, Ketelson, SM, Weaver, CM and Erdman, JW Jr (1986). Bioavailability

of zinc to rats as affected by protein source and previous dietary intake. *J Nutr*, **116**, 1423–1431

173. Van Barneveld, AA and VandenHamer, CJA (1985). Influence of isotope administration mode and of food consumption on absorption and retention of ^{65}Zn in mice. *Nutr Rept Int*, **31**, 887–894

174. Becker, WM and Hoekstra, WG (1971). The intestinal absorption of zinc. In Skoryna, SC and Waldron-Edward, D (eds), *Intestinal Absorption of Metal Ions, Trace Elements and Radionuclides*, pp. 229–256 (New York: Pergamon Press)

175. Minami, H and McCallum, RW (1984). The physiology and pathophysiology of gastric emptying in humans. *Gastroenterology*, **86**, 1592–1610

176. Malagelada, J-R (1981). Gastric, pancreatic, and biliary responses to a meal. In Johnson, LR (ed), *Physiology of the Gastrointestinal Tract*, pp. 893–924 (New York: Raven Press)

177. Malagelada, J-R, Go, LWV and Summerskill, WHJ (1979). Different gastric, pancreatic, and biliary responses to solid–liquid or homogenized meals. *Dig Dis Sci*, **24**, 101–110

178. Nowak, A, Jonderko, K, Kaczor, R *et al.* (1987). Cigarette smoking delays gastric emptying of a radiolabelled solid food in healthy smokers. *Scand J Gastroenterol*, **22**, 54–58

179. Hunt, JR, Johnson, PE and Swan, PB (1987). Dietary conditions influencing relative zinc availability from foods to the rat, and correlations with *in vitro* measurements. *J Nutr* **117**, 1913–1923

180. Hunt, JR, Johnson, PE and Swan, PB (1987). The effect of dietary zinc before and after ^{65}Zn administration on absorption and turnover of ^{65}Zn. *Trace Elements in Man and Animals (TEMA-6)* (in press)

181. Neathery, MW, Lassiter, JW, Miller, WJ and Gentry, RP (1975). Absorption, excretion, and tissue distribution of natural organic and inorganic ^{65}Zn in the rat. *Proc Soc Exp Biol Med*, **149**, 1–4

182. Evans, GW and Johnson, PE (1977). Determination of zinc availability in foods by the extrinsic label technique. *Am J Clin Nutr*, **30**, 873–878

183. Meyer, NR, Stuart, MA and Weaver, CM (1983). Bioavailability of zinc from defatted soy flour, soy hulls and whole eggs as determined by intrinsic and extrinsic labeling techniques. *J Nutr*, **113**, 1255–1264

184. Ketelsen, SM, Stuart, MA, Weaver, CM *et al.* (1984). Bioavailability of zinc to rats from defatted soy flour, acid-precipitated soy concentrate and neutralized soy concentrate as determined by intrinsic and extrinsic labeling techniques. *J Nutr*, **114**, 536–542

185. Sandström, B, Keen, CL and Lönnerdal, B (1983). An experimental model for studies of zinc bioavailability from milk and infant formulas using extrinsic labeling. *Am J Clin Nutr*, **38**, 20–428

186. Janghorbani, M, Istfan, NW, Pagounes, JO *et al.* (1982). Absorption of dietary zinc in man: comparison of intrinsic and extrinsic labels using a triple stable isotope method. *Am J Clin Nutr*, **36**, 537–545

187. Flanagan, PR, Cluett, J, Chamberlain, MJ and Valberg, LS (1985). Dual-isotope method for determination of human zinc absorption: the use of a test meal of turkey meat. *J Nutr*, **115**, 111–122

188. Johnson, PE, Mahalko, JR, Gallaher, DD *et al.* (1986). Absorption of ^{65}Zn by humans fed intrinsically and extrinsically labeled beef. *J Nutr*, **116**, xliii

189. Song, MK, Adham, NF and Ament, ME (1985). A possible role of zinc on the intestinal calcium absorption mechanisms in rats. *Nutr Rept Int*, **31**, 43–51

190. Sandström, B and Cederblad, Å (1980). Zinc absorption from composite meals. II. Influence of the main protein source. *Am J Clin Nutr*, **33**, 1778–1783

191. Solomons, NW, Pineda, O, Viteri, F and Sandstead, HH (1983). Studies on the

bioavailability of zinc in humans: mechanism of the intestinal interaction of non heme iron and zinc. *J Nutr*, 113, 337–349

192. Sandström, B, Davidsson, L, Cederblad, Å, Lönnerdal, B (1985). Oral iron, dietary ligands and zinc absorption. *J Nutr*, 115, 411–414

193. Valberg, LS, Flanagan, PR and Chamberlain, MJ (1984). Effects of iron, tin, and copper on zinc absorption in humans. *Am J Clin Nutr*, 40, 536–541

194. Van Campen, DR (1969). Copper interference with the intestinal absorption of ^{65}Zn by rats. *J Nutr*, 97, 104–108

195. Milne, DB, Canfield, WK, Mahalko, JR and Sandstead, HH (1984). Effect of oral folic acid supplements on zinc, copper, and iron absorption and excretion. *Am J Clin Nutr*, 39, 535–539

196. Evans, GW and Johnson, EC (1981). Effect of iron, vitamin B-6 and picolinic acid on zinc absorption in the rat. *J Nutr*, 111, 68–75

197. Solomons, NW, Janghorbani, M, Ting, BTG *et al.* (1982). Bioavailability of zinc from a diet based on isolated soy protein: application in young men of the stable isotope tracer, ^{70}Zn. *J Nutr*, 112, 1809–1821

198. Van Campen, D and House, WA (1974). Effect of a low protein diet on retention of an oral dose of ^{65}Zn and on tissue concentrations of zinc, iron, and copper in rats. *J Nutr*, 104, 84–90

199. Snedeker, SM and Greger, JL (1983). Metabolism of zinc, copper and iron as affected by dietary protein, cysteine and histidine. *J Nutr*, 113, 644–652

200. Young, VR and Janghorbani, M (1982). Legumes and mineral absorption, with special reference to soybean proteins. *J Plan Foods*, 4, 57–73

201. Welch, RM and House, WA (1982). Availability to rats of zinc from soybean seeds as affected by maturity of seed, source of dietary protein, and soluble phytate. *J Nutr*, 112, 879–885

202. Lo, GS, Settle, SL, Steinke, FH and Hopkins, DT (1981). Effect of phytate: zinc molar ratio and isolated soybean protein zinc bioavailability. *J Nutr*, 111, 2223–2235

203. Sandström, B, Kivisto, B and Cederblad, Å (1987). Absorption of zinc from soy protein meals in humans. *J Nutr*, 117, 321–327

204. Auge, M, Kreiling, R, Harzer, G, Daniel, H and Rehner, G (1986). Effect of proteins on availability of zinc. II. Bioavailability of zinc from casein and whey protein-retention study in young rats. *Z Ernährgswiss*, 25, 233–241

205. O'Dell, BL, Burpo, DE and Savage, JE (1972). Evaluation of zinc availability in foodstuffs of plant and animal origin. *J Nutr*, 102, 653–660

206. Prasad, AS, Miale, A, Farid, Z *et al.* (1963). Zinc metabolism in patients with the syndrome of iron deficiency anemia, hypogonadism, and dwarfism. *J Lab Clin Med*, 61, 537–549

207. Davies, NT and Nightingale, R (1975). The effects of phytate on intestinal absorption and secretion of zinc, and whole-body retention of Zn, copper, iron and manganese in rats. *Br J Nutr* 34, 243–258

208. Anonymous (1983). Phytate and zinc metabolism. *Nutr Rev*, 41, 64–66

209. Morris, ER and Ellis, R (1980). Bioavailability to rats of iron and zinc in wheat bran: response to low-phytate bran and effect of the phytate/zinc molar ratio. *J Nutr*, 110, 2000–2010

210. Navert, B, Sandström, B and Cederblad, Å (1985). Reduction of the phytate content of bran by leavening in bread and its effect on zinc absorption in man. *Br J Nutr*, 53, 47–53

211. Turnlund, JR, King, JC, Keyes, WR *et al.* (1984). A stable isotope study of zinc absorption in young men: effects of phytate and cellulose. *Am J Clin Nutr*, 40, 1071–1077

212. Sandberg, A-S, Hasselblad, C, Hasselblad, K and Hulten, L (1982). The effect of wheat bran on the absorption of minerals in the small intestine. *Br J Nutr*, 48, 185–191

213. Reinhold, JG, Faradji, B, Abadi, P and Ismael-Beigi, F (1976). Decreased absorption of calcium, magnesium, zinc and phosphorus by humans due to increased fiber and phosphorus consultion as wheat bread. *J Nutr*, **106**, 493–503

214. Bagheri, SM and Guéguen, L (1982). Effects of wheat bran on the metabolism of ^{45}Ca and ^{65}Zn in rats. *J Nutr*, **112**, 2047–2051

215. Van Dokkum, W, Wesstra, A and Schippers, FA (1982). Physiological effects of fibre-rich types of bread. 1. The effect of dietary fibre from bread on the mineral balance of young men. *Br J Nutr*, **47**, 451–460

216. Caprez, A and Fairweather-Tait, SJ (1982). The effect of heat treatment and particle size of bran on mineral absorption in rats. *Br J Nutr*, **48**, 467

217. Welch, RM, House, WA and Van Campen, D (1977). Effects of oxalic acid on availability of zinc from spinach leaves and zinc sulfate to rats. *J Nutr*, **7**, 929

218. McDonald, JT and Margen, S (1980). Wine versus ethanol in human nutrition. IV. Zinc balance. *Am J Clin Nutr*, **33**, 1096–1102

219. Atonson, DL and Vanderhoof, JA (1983). Effect of chronic ethanol ingestion on zinc absorption in rat small intestine. *Dig Dis Sci*, **28**, 604–608

220. Ahmed, SB and Russell, RM (1982). The effect of ethanol feeding on zinc balance and tissue zinc levels in rats maintained on zinc deficient diets. *J Lab Clin Med*, **100**, 211–217

10
Concerning the potential therapeutic value of zinc in rheumatoid and psoriatic arthritis

A Frigo, LM Bambara, E Concari*, M Marrella*, U Moretti*,
C Tambalo, GP Velo* and R Milanino*
Istituto di Patologia Medica and Istituto di Farmacologia*, Università di
Verona, Policlinico Borgo Roma, 37134 Verona, Italy

I. RHEUMATOID ARTHRITIS (RA)

(1) Zinc status

Although less extensively studied than copper, the metabolism of zinc has also been shown to be affected by rheumatoid arthritic conditions, a decrease of plasma zinc concentration being the change most frequently observed.

Niedermeier and Griggs[1] have reported a significant decrease of plasma zinc values in 68 RA patients, and found high levels of zinc, copper and iron in the synovial fluids of most of them. Sorenson and Di Tommaso[2] measured a 40% decrease of serum zinc concentration in RA patients whose serum Mg levels were found to be normal; on the basis of these observations the authors concluded that the fall of circulating zinc was a feature of rheumatoid arthritis rather than an epiphenomenon due to malabsorption possibly associated with the disease itself. Balogh and co-workers[3] found a reduced plasma zinc concentration in RA patients, and showed that plasma zinc was directly correlated to serum albumin and inversely correlated to erythrocyte sedimentation rate (ESR) and serum globulins. These authors failed, however, to find a significant correlation between plasma zinc levels and the number of tender joints or rheumatoid factor. In another study the reduced plasma zinc concentration measured in RA patients was found to be significantly correlated with the duration but not with the severity of the disease[4].

Zinc concentration in the peripheral blood cells has been recently studied by Svenson and co-workers[5], who found values lower than normal in patients with rheumatoid arthritis and other inflammatory connective tissue diseases.

Copper and Zinc in Inflammation. Milanino, R, Rainsford, KD and Velo, GP (eds)
Inflammation and Drug Therapy Series, Volume IV

The urinary output of zinc may also be influenced by rheumatoid arthritis. An increase of urinary excretion of zinc in RA patients was indeed reported by some authors[6-8], but not confirmed by others[9].

In our laboratory we have in preliminary studies examined the plasma concentration as well as the urinary excretion of zinc in 54 patients with established rheumatoid arthritis. The results obtained (Table 1) have shown a statistically significant decrease of plasma zinc, whereas no changes were observed in the amounts of metal measured in the 24 h urine. Most interestingly, however, we found a statistically significant correlation between plasma zinc levels and some relevant markers of the disease such as duration of the illness, ESR values, number of swollen joints, etc. (Table 2).

Table 1 Plasma and 24 h urine zinc status in normal individuals and in patients with rheumatoid arthritis and osteoarthrosis (osteoarthritis)

Group	n	Plasma zinc μg/dl (SD)	Urinary zinc μg/24 h (SD)
Normal	29	106 (22)	458 (274)
Osteoarthritis	18	104 (13)	476 (216)
Rheumatoid arthritis	54	97 (15)*	451 (208)

The normal group (comprising healthy hospital personnel) was selected to have mean age and sex distribution comparable to those found in the RA group. Zinc determination were made by flame atomic absorption spectroscopy[22].
* $p < 0.010$, Student's t-test versus normal group.

Table 2 Rheumatoid arthritis: correlation coefficients (r) between plasma zinc concentration values and some classical parameters characterizing the disease status

Parameter	r	p
Duration of the illness	−0.43	< 0.001
Number of swollen joints	−0.35	< 0.050
Erythrocyte sedimentation rate (ESR)	−0.44	< 0.001
α_2–globulins	−0.34	< 0.050
Haemoglobin	0.30	< 0.050

Finally, the relevance of the anti-arthritic therapy on the zinc status in RA patients has been scarcely investigated, and very few data are, at present, available. Corticosteroid treatment seemed to exacerbate the plasma zinc deficiency observed in RA patients[4], whereas D-penicillamine has been found to significantly increase the concentration of zinc in plasma and erythrocytes, as well as the amount of zinc in the 24 h urine of rheumatoid patients[10]. Gold therapy is capable of inducing an increase of hepatic and renal zinc and metallothionein levels in the rat[11] and thus may be assumed to interfere with the zinc status of RA patients. In our hands, however, the plasma zinc concentrations of 11 RA patients treated with gold preparations

(99.9 ± 11.9 μg/dl) was found to be comparable to that observed in the whole population of RA patients examined (97.0 ± 15.0 μg/dl).

(2) Zinc therapy

Simkin[12] was the first to carry out a controlled trial orally administering zinc sulphate (220 mg three times daily) to a group of 24 middle-aged RA patients, most of whom had active disease of long duration. The author described the rationale of this study as follows: (1) rheumatoid arthritis may be characterized by a zinc-deficiency status; (2) the efficacy of D-penicillamine in the therapy of RA conditions may be partly due to its ability in promoting intestinal zinc absorption; (3) zinc may have anti-inflammatory properties *in vivo* being, *in vitro* capable of stabilizing lysosomal membranes as well as modulating complement and macrophages activities. Of the 21 RA patients out of the 24 initially enrolled, all completed the trial showing a statistically significant improvement in joint swelling, severity of morning stiffness, 50-foot walking time and patients' overall impression of their well-being. In addition, patients tolerated oral zinc sulphate well, leading Simkin to suggest that zinc therapy deserves further study in active RA conditions. According to Simkin[13], zinc therapy was also successful in ameliorating significantly joint swelling, joint tenderness, 50-foot walking time, morning stiffness, onset of fatigue and global impression of general condition in 18 RA patients quoted as having been studied in India by Dr Desai and colleagues.

Two later studies, however, failed to confirm the above observations. Mattingly and Mowat[14], in a double-blind trial versus placebo conducted on 27 RA patients, examined the efficacy of zinc sulphate (220 mg three times daily) in controlling active rheumatoid arthritis. After 6 months of oral therapy no differences, either on clinical and laboratory ground, were seen between zinc- and placebo-treated patients. Similar results were also reported by Rasker and Kardaun[15] in an open trial on 22 patients affected by rheumatoid arthritis refractory to gold salt, D-penicillamine and anti-malarial therapies. Cousins and Swerdel[16] have recently shown that the parenteral administration of zinc sulphate is capable of reducing the inflammatory response inducing, at the same time, a further increase of serum caeruloplasmin levels in treated compared with non-treated adjuvant arthritic rats, a representative animal model of human rheumatoid arthritis. These latter observations may perhaps suggest further study of the potential therapeutic value of zinc in RA conditions.

II. PSORIATIC ARTHRITIS (PA)

(1) Zinc status

In the late 1960s plasma zinc concentration was evaluated in psoriatic patients and found to be normal by one group[17], and decreased by another two groups[18],[19] of researchers. The problem of plasma zinc levels in psoriatic patients was more recently re-examined by McMillan and co-workers[20], who observed a decreased concentration of circulating metal ion, also showing a statistically significant inverse correlation between plasma zinc and the extent of cutaneous lesion. Clemmensen and co-workers[21] found plasma zinc concentration to be within normal range in patients with psoriatic arthritis accompanied by mild psoriasis. In our laboratory we have done a preliminary examination of zinc status, as well as the copper status, in 20 patients with active psoriatic arthritis accompanied by a mild to moderate extent of cutaneous lesions. The results obtained are summarized in Table 3. Although lower than normal, plasma zinc concentration was not significantly different compared with that of healthy controls, whereas plasma copper levels proved to be statistically significantly increased. No differences were observed, for either copper and zinc, in the cell fraction of blood (Table 3) or in the urinary excretion of metal ions (data not shown).

Table 3 Copper and zinc status in blood control subjects and PA patients

| Group | n | BLOOD COPPER | | BLOOD ZINC | |
		Plasma µg/dl (SD)	Cells µg/dl of blood (SD)	Plasma µg/dl (SD)	Cells µg/dl of blood SD)
Healthy blood donors	30	113 (14)	39.9 (4.9)	108 (10)	633 (66)
PA patients	20	141 (31)*	39.5 (4.6)	101 (22)	621 (86)

The control group (healthy blood donors) was selected to have mean age and sex distribution comparable to those found in the PA patient group. Copper and zinc determinations were made by flame atomic absorption spectroscopy according to a previously published procedure[22].
* $p < 0.001$; Student's t-test versus healthy blood donors.

According to the above data, the lack of hypozincaemia might be taken as a further parameter differentiating psoriatic from rheumatoid arthritis, provided that the former is not associated with severe cutaneous lesions.

(2) Zinc therapy

Clemmensen and co-workers[21] were the first, and to our knowledge the only, group that has attempted to use zinc as a therapeutic agent in PA conditions. Twenty-four patients with active psoriatic arthritis were admitted to a double-blind cross-over trial carried out with oral zinc sulphate (220 mg three times daily) versus placebo. In this study, after the first 6 weeks the zinc-treated patients moved to placebo while the placebo-treated patients moved to zinc for a second 6-week period. At the end of this first study, statistical significance was attained only for the improvements recorded in joint pain and non-steroidal anti-inflammatory drug (NSAID) consumption. The patients were then enrolled in a further 6-month open trial with zinc sulphate. During this period morning stiffness, overall condition, joint tenderness and

136

motility all appeared to improve significantly. Moreover, serum albumin increased and serum immunoglobulin decreased. The therapy did not modify the extent of patients' cutaneous lesions. The authors concluded that oral zinc sulphate may well be beneficial in psoriatic arthritis.

Encouraged by the above observations we decided to undertake a preliminary uncontrolled study in Verona. Twenty patients (14 males and 6 females; mean age 48.4 years) affected by mild to moderate psoriasis and active psoriatic arthritis (mono-arthritis in 2, oligoarthritis in 6 and poly-arthritis in 12 cases) whose duration ranged from 0.5 to 20 years, were enrolled in a 6-month open trial with oral zinc sulphate (200 mg three times daily, equivalent to 120 mg/day of elemental zinc). Seventeen of the 20 patients were treated with symptomatic drugs (13 with NSAIDs, 3 with NSAIDs plus corticosteroids, 1 with corticosteroids only), whereas none of them had been treated with any disease-modifying antirheumatic drug during the year preceding the beginning of the trial.

Two of the 20 patients were withdrawn from the trial because of gastric intolerance to the drug, while another eight recorded mild nausea and constipation, both of which regressed upon continuation of therapy. The remainder tolerated zinc treatment very well.

The 18 patients who completed the trial showed, at the 6-month control (see Table 4), a statistically significant decrease in the number of both swollen ($p < 0.050$) and tender ($p < 0.010$) joints as well as a significant reduction in Ritchie's index ($p < 0.010$) and of NSAID consumption ($p < 0.001$). The final global evaluation of physician and patient concordantly recorded two patients asymptomatic, 14 patients very improved or improved, and 2 patients stationary. By the end of the trial 11 of 18 PA patients have completely stopped the symptomatic therapy. The laboratory parameters (Table 5) showed, in addition to an increase above normal of plasma zinc values, a statistically significant decrease of ESR ($p < 0.001$), and a decrease of plasma copper ($p < 0.001$ at 6 months) whose levels, by the end of the trial, were found comparable to those measured in the healthy controls (Table 3). No statistically significant changes were observed in the blood-cell copper or zinc status (Table 5), or in urinary copper excretion (data not shown). Conversely, zinc levels in the 24 h urine dramatically increased by a factor ranging from 3 to 4 (data not shown). The therapy did not modify the extent of patients' cutaneous lesions.

After the trial a group of 11 patients continued the follow-up, which continued for over a year. Within this group 4 patients achieved remission, while 3 who were classified as improved at the end of the trial are still in very good overall condition with no changes since last visit and no need of symptomatic drugs. The arthritis deteriorated in 5 patients following withdrawal of zinc treatment. Three of these patients were submitted to one or two more 6-month cycles with oral zinc sulphate, again obtaining good clinical improvement, while the other 2 patients resumed the symptomatic treatment. Finally, 1 patient, who was judged improved at the end of the trial, was placed on

Table 4 Some major clinical parameters during ZnSO$_4$ therapy in 18 PA patients

Parameter	Basal values x (SD)	Months of therapy 2 x (SD)	4 x (SD)	6 x (SD)
Tender joints	13.4 (7.7)	7.5 (4.3)**	6.4 (4.6)**	7.2 (4.6)**
Swollen joints	4.3 (3.1)	2.8 (3.1)	2.3 (2.7)*	1.9 (2.7)*
Ritchie's index	12.4 (7.4)	6.8 (3.5)**	5.3 (3.5)***	5.4 (3.9)**
Morning stiffness (min)	35.8 (42.6)	16.4 (28.3)	13.1 (28.3)	15.0 (33.3)
Grip strength (mmHg)	165.1 (89.0)	180.9 (85.2)	195.2 (81.4)	184.9 (81.1)
NSAID consumption[a]	14.3 (5.4)	7.1 (7.0)**	2.6 (4.3)***	1.8 (3.5)***

*$p < 0.050$, **$p < 0.010$, ***$p < 0.001$, Student's t test versus basal values.
[a]Number of non-steroidal anti-inflammatory drug tablets weekly consumed.

Table 5   Trend of some major laboratory parameters during ZnSO₄ therapy in 18 PA patients

Parameter (units)	Basal values x (SD)	Months of therapy 2 x (SD)	4 x (SD)	6 x (SD)
ESR (mm/h)	36.9 (27.5)	27.2 (25.2)	23.1 (15.5)	10.1 (9.3)***
C-reactive protein (mg/dl)	2.3 (3.5)	0.7 (0.8)	0.4 (0.8)*	0.6 (1.2)
α_2-globulins (%)	10.3 (2.3)	9.5 (2.3)	8.8 (1.5)*	9.3 (2.3)
γ-globulins (%)	18.6 (5.0)	17.3 (4.3)	18.8 (4.6)	17.5 (4.3)
Fibrinogen (mg/dl)	432.1 (190.1)	409.0 (177.9)	361.2 (97.4)	348.3 (89.2)
Plasma Cu (μg/dl)	141.2 (30.9)	121.1 (21.0)*	119.9 (17.4)*	111.0 (13.0)***
Blood cell Cu (μg/dl)	39.5 (4.6)	39.6 (7.7)	38.5 (7.0)	37.5 (6.8)
Plasma Zn (μg/dl)	101.0 (22.4)	153.2 (36.1)***	164.1 (37.0)***	151.9 (46.1)***
Blood cell Zn (μg/dl)	621.1 (86.2)	606.4 (100.2)	632.3 (90.1)	648.7 (107.6)

Copper and zinc determinations were made by flame atomic absorption spectroscopy according to a previously published procedure[22].
* $p < 0.050$, *** $p < 0.001$; Student's t-test basal values.

gold-salt therapy. After 1 year of gold treatment her overall condition was found unchanged, and no further improvement was observed compared to the results obtained with the previous zinc therapy.

In conclusion, the results summarized above may further suggest that peroral zinc sulphate treatment is effective in controlling the articular symptomatology due to to PA conditions, possibly acting as a disease-modifying antirheumatic agent. In our hands a significant improvement of clinical, as well as laboratory, parameters directly related to disease activity was observed in over 80% of treated PA patients, and although the possibility of a placebo effect cannot be neglected, some relevant evidence seems to contradict this hypothesis. This includes: the very high percentage of improved patients; the extent of improvement itself, as well as its lasting beyond the withdrawal of therapy; and, especially, the ESR values of PA patients found to be dramatically (–70%) and highly significantly ($p < 0.001$) reduced by the zinc treatment. In our opinion it is unlikely that the observed results are casually related to the natural cyclic evolution of the studied disease. Indeed, the follow-up carried out after the trial showed five patients to relapse and three out these to improve again upon zinc sulphate therapy resumption.

Further work is in progress to verify more strictly, in a double-blind cross-over 1-year trial versus placebo, the efficacy of oral zinc in the treatment of psoriatic arthritis.

III. CONCLUDING REMARKS

The results summarized in this paper, although certainly not conclusive, redirect attention to the use of zinc in the therapy of inflammatory chronic autoimmune diseases such as rheumatoid and psoriatic arthritis. The very low toxicity of zinc preparations – especially in comparison to that exhibited by NSAIDs and by disease-modifying antirheumatic agents like gold salts, D-penicillamine or levamisole – may be a further relevant reason encouraging such a novel approach. Amongst the side-effects produced by zinc administration, however, is the possibility that prolonged use of oral zinc may eventually induce some degree of copper deficiency, inhibiting the intestinal absorption of this latter trace element. Such an effect would be especially unwelcome since a dietary or environmental-induced copper deficiency has been suggested, in man, to be a contributory factor in the aetiology of arthritic conditions[23]. Thus zinc inhibits intestinal copper absorption in the rat[24], and this influence has been successfully exploited in the treatment of Wilson's disease[25,26]. In man not affected by inherited disturbances of copper metabolism, however, an excessive oral intake of zinc (150–450 mg/day, taken for 2 years) was found to promote a copper-deficiency status revealed by hypocupraemia and hypocaeruloplasminaemia, and associated anaemia usually of the hypochromic microcytic type[27–29]. According to Prasad and co-workers[27] this condition was easily corrected by oral copper supplementation. Much lower doses of oral zinc, in healthy adult men, failed to produce either hypocupraemia or anaemia, but were shown to reduce the retention of dietary copper following 2 weeks on 18.5 mg/day zinc administration[30], and to slightly, yet significantly, decrease the erythrocyte Cu, Zn-superoxide dismutase (SOD) activity after 6 weeks on a 50 mg/day zinc dosage[31].

In our hands the 18 PA patients taking 120 mg/day of oral zinc for at least 6 months did not show any sign of anaemia and, although erythrocyte SOD activity has not been measured, the copper concentration in the cell fraction of blood was found to be substantially unaffected by zinc therapy (note that over 60% of total erythrocyte copper is bound to SOD[32]). As reported above, we found the plasma copper levels to be significantly decreased in treated PA patients who were hypercupraemic before therapy. At the present time we do not know whether this latter result has been induced by an inhibition of copper absorption, by the success of oral zinc therapy, or possibly by both. In our opinion all available evidence may suggest carefully following the copper status in patients undergoing chronic or prolonged oral zinc treatment, to ascertain possible need for copper supplements.

References

1. Niedermeier, W and Grigge, JH (1971). Trace metal composition of synovial fluid and blood serum of patients with rheumatoid arthritis. *J Chron Dis*, 23, 527–36
2. Sorenson, JRJ and Di Tommaso, DJ (1977). Mean serum copper, magnesium and zinc concentration in active rheumatoid and other degenerative connective tissue disease. In Hemphill, DD (ed.), *Trace Substances in Environmental Health*, Vol. XI (Columbia: University of Missouri), pp. 15–22
3. Balogh, Z, El-Gobarey, AF, Fell, GS *et al.* (1980). Plasma zinc and its relationship to clinical symptoms and drug treatment in rheumatoid arthritis. *Ann Rheum Dis*, 39, 329–32
4. Morgenstern, H and Machtey, I (1983). Serum zinc and copper levels in rheumatoid arthritis. *Arthritis Rheum*, 26, 933–4
5. Svenson, KLG, Hallgren, R, Johansson, E and Lindth, U (1985). Reduced zinc in peripheral blood cells from patients with inflammatory connective tissue diseases. *Inflammation*, 9, 189–99
6. Pandey, SP, Bhattacharya, SK and Sundar, S (1985). Zinc in rheumatoid arthritis. *Indian J Med Res*, 81, 618–20
7. Bonebrake, RA, McCall, JT, Hunder, GG and Polley, HF (1972). Zinc accumulation in synovial fluid. *Mayo Clin Proc*, 47, 746–50
8. Ambanelli, U, Ferraccioli, GF, Bernardi, P and Serventi, G (1978). Relation between urine zinc and hydroxyproline in rheumatoid arthritis and bone disease. *J Rheumatol*, 5, 477–9
9. Aaseth, J, Munthe, E, Forre, O and Steinnes, E (1978). Trace elements in serum and urine of patients with rheumatoid arthritis. *Scand J Rheumatol*, 7, 237–40
10. Jepsen, LV and Pedersen, KH (1984). Changes in zinc and zinc-dependent enzymes in rheumatoid patients during penicillamine treatment. *Scand J Rheumatol*, 13, 282–8
11. Sharma, RP (1983). Metabolism of intracellular zinc and copper following single and repeated injections of gold sodium thiomalate. *Agents and Actions*, 14, 380–8
12. Simkin, PA (1976). Oral zinc sulphate in rheumatoid arthritis. *Lancet*, 2, 539–42

13. Simkin, PA (1982). Treatment of rheumatoid arthritis with zinc sulphate. In *Inflammatory Disease and Copper*, ed. Sorenson, JRJ (Clifton, New Jersey: Humana Press), pp. 483–93

14. Mattingly, PC and Mowat, AG (1982). Zinc sulphate in rheumatoid arthritis. *Ann Rheum Dis*, **41**, 456–7

15. Rasker, JJ and Kardaun, SH (1982). Lack of beneficial effect of zinc sulphate in rheumatoid arthritis. *Scand J Rheumatol*, **11**, 168–70

16. Cousins, RJ and Swerdel, MR (1985). Ceruloplasmin and metallothionein induction by zinc and 13-cis-retinoic acid in rats with adjuvant inflammation. *Proc Soc Exp Biol Med*, **179**, 168–72

17. Withers, AFD, Baker, H, Musa, M and Dormandy, TL (1968). Plasma zinc in psoriasis. *Lancet*, **2**, 278

18. Greaves, MW and Boyde, TRC (1967). Plasma zinc concentration in patients with psoriasis, other dermatoses and venous leg ulcerations. *Lancet*, **2**, 1019

19. Voorhees, JJ, Chakrabarti, SE, Botero, E *et al.* (1969). Zinc therapy and distribution in psoriasis. *Arch Dermatol*, **100**, 669

20. McMillan, EM and Rowe, D (1983). Plasma zinc in psoriasis: relation to surface area involvement. *Br J Dermatol*, **108**, 301–5

21. Clemmensen, OJ, Siggard-Andersen, J, Worm, AM *et al.* (1980). Psoriasis treated with oral zinc sulphate. *Br J Dermatol*, **103**, 411–5

22. Marella, M and Milanino, R (1986). Simple and reproducible method for extraction of copper and zinc from rat tissue for determination by flame atomic absorption spectroscopy. *Atomic Spectrosc*, **7**, 40–2

23. Rainsford, KD (1982). Environmental metal ion perturbations, especially as they affect copper status, are a factor in the etiology of arthritic conditions: an hypothesis. In *Inflammatory Diseases and Copper*, (ed.) Sorenson, JRJ (Clifton, New Jersey: Humana Press), pp. 137–43

24. Oestreicher, P and Cousins, RJ (1985). Copper and zinc absorption in the rat: mechanism of mutual antagonism. *J Nutr*, **115**, 159–66

25. Brewer, GJ, Hill, GM, Prasad, AS *et al.* (1983). Oral zinc therapy for Wilson's disease. *Ann Intern Med*, **99**, 314–20

26. Hoogenraad, TU, Van den Hamer, CJ and Van Hattum, J (1984). Effective treatment of Wilson's disease with oral zinc sulphate: two case reports. *Br Med J*, **289**, 273–6

27. Prasad, AS, Brewer, GJ, Schoomaker, EB and Rabbani, P (1978). Hypocupremia induced by zinc therapy in adults. *J Am Med Assoc*, **240**, 2166–8

28. Anonymous (1985). Copper deficiency induced by megadoses of zinc. *Nutr Rev*, **43**, 148–9

29. Patterson, WP, Winkelmann, M and Perry, MC (1985). Zinc-induced copper deficiency: megamineral sideroblastic anemia. *Ann Intern Med*, **103**, 385–6

30. Festa, MD, Anderson, HL, Dowdy, RP and Ellersieck, MR (1985). Effect of zinc intake on copper excretion and retention in man. *Am J Clin Nutr*, **41**, 285–92

31. Fischer, PWF, Giroux, A and L'Abbè, MR (1984). Effect of zinc supplementation on copper status in adult man. *Am J Clin Nutr*, **40**, 743–6

32. Underwood, EJ (1977). *Trace Elements in Human and Animal Nutrition*, (New York: Academic Press), pp. 56–108

Index

absorption
  of topically applied copper complexes,
    89, 90
  zinc, 103–21
    effects of food/food components on,
      118–21
    effects of testing conditions on, 116–17
    methods of assessment, 113–18
    physiological factors affecting, 112–13
    process of, 103–9
acetate, copper complexes of,
    anti-inflammatory activity, 74, 75
acrodermatitis enteropathica, treatment,
    107–8
adjuvant arthritis, anti-inflammatory
    activity of copper complexes in,
    75, 88, 90–1
albumin
  antioxidant activity, 14
  copper complexes with, 10
    in rheumatoid arthritis, 10
alcoholic drinks, zinc absorption and the
    effects of, 120–1
Alcusal®, 85–6
amine oxidases, function, 71
amino acid(s), zinc transport involving, 106,
    107–8
amino acid-copper complexes, free radical
    scavenging, 53–4
cAMP, metallothionein inducibility by, 24,
    26
anaemia, zinc therapy-related, 140–1
analgesic activities of copper complexes,
    76, 77
ankylosing spondylitis, copper studies in, 3
anti-inflammatory activities of
    copper/copper compounds, 52,
    54–5, 74–6, 88, 90–1, 98–101
antioxidant copper proteins, see copper
    proteins
anti-ulcer activities of copper complexes,
    78–81
apocaeruloplasmin, copper incorporation
    into, 25, 26
apometalloenzymes, copper and zinc
    donation to, 26
arthritis

adjuvant, anti-inflammatory activity of
    copper complexes in, 75, 88, 90–1
  psoriatic, see psoriatic arthritis
  rheumatoid, see rheumatoid arthritis
ascorbic acid levels in rheumatoid arthritis,
    13
aspirin
  copper complexes and,
    anti-inflammatory activity of,
    comparison, 75
  copper complexes of
    analgesic activity, 76, 77
    anti-inflammatory activity, 75
    anti-ulcer activity, 79, 80
    toxicity studies, 75, 76

beverages, zinc absorption and the effects
    of, 120–1
bile, copper content, 69
biodistribution of copper from topically
    applied copper complexes, 88–90
bis(2-benzyimidazoylyl)thioether ligands,
    95–101
bis(glycinato) copper complexes, skin
    permeation by, 85
bleomycin, catalytic iron and copper assays
    employing, 10
blood cells, peripheral, in inflammatory
    diseases, zinc concentrations in,
    133, see also specific cell types
bone
  resorption, copper-inhibited, 54
  zinc incoporation into, zinc
    bioavailability determined via, 116
bone marrow
  progenitor cells, metallothionein
    expression in, 26
  zinc in, metabolically active nature of, 26
bread, dietary, zinc absorption and the
    effects of, 120
brush border membrane vesicles, zinc
    transport studies using, 105
brush border proteins, zinc transport
    involving, 106

caeruloplasmin, 3–4, 13–17, see also
    apocaeruloplasmin

143